Danger: I'm A Nurse With A Penis

Stories And Lessons From The Field

By Walt Cummings

© 2018 by Walt Cummings

All rights reserved. This book or any portion thereof may not be reproduced or used in any manner whatsoever without the express written permission of the publisher except for the use of brief quotations in a book review.

Printed in the United States of America

First Printing, 2018

nursewaltcummings@gmail.com

ISBN: 9781717713285

www.malenurseblog.com

Ejaculation: this book is a work of fiction designed to entertain you. I am a nurse in real life and want to share with you some experiences as a male nurse.

Prologue	5
Chapter 1: I Should Have Been a Doctor	8
Chapter 2: Why Am I Taking Orders From a Woman?	13
Chapter 3: How To Survive The Night Shift	17
Chapter 4: I Want to Smash My Classmates	23
Chapter 5: I Want To Be A CRNA	29
Chapter 6: Disciplinary Action And Getting Fired	36
Chapter 7: Dipping Your Hand In Shit	59
Chapter 8: How To Go To School For Free	64
Chapter 9: How To Leave Nursing And Get Owned	74
Chapter 10: The Sunk Cost Fallacy	80

Prologue

Most books about men in nursing are full of shit. I've tried to minimize the amount of bullshit in this book.

I want to tell you ten different stories as a male nurse that are both extreme and true (none of them will be about guys fucking each other, since 90% of guys in nursing are straight). Worst case is that you get entertained. Best case is that you learn something. Either way, you win.

I also want to reveal the struggles of male nurses and the ways to cope with them. Through a series of ten stories, I hope to make the journey as a male nurse a little easier.

How did this book come to be? When I was an 18 year old undergraduate at NYU, I was lost. During the second night of orientation, I realized that the status of my school meant nothing. The students around me were obsessing over meaningless things, such as frat parties and the football team. Amid this teenage confusion, I thought to myself: "what's the real point of going to college? Isn't it to get a job?" In my hopelessness as a Psychobiology student with no job prospects, I decided to commit to a career in nursing.

I ended up with a nursing job. I worked for a couple of years in critical care and then enrolled in CRNA school (CRNA=nurse who gives anesthesia). I was seduced by how easy the role of the CRNA seemed. However, the prospect of paying $140,000 was so daunting that I woke up one night at 2 am in abject terror. I knew I had to take massive action to avoid the huge debt load, so I decided to commit myself to 30 minutes a day of scholarship writing. By consistently applying for scholarships everyday, I was able to win some cash. Little did I know that the school would ask me to withdraw one year after classes started (continue reading for the juicy story). In the process of withdrawing from CRNA school, I discovered that I should just stick to writing. All that said, this handbook is a byproduct of my journey to CRNA school. My CRNA dream didn't work out, but I learned valuable lessons along the way.

The male nurse journey, especially for guys in their twenties, is very tough. You will feel like quitting many times. You will also think countless times that the grass is greener on the other side, whether that side be pharmacy, dentistry, or medicine. At the same time, you will cry, you will laugh, and you will say "wow" more times than you thought possible.

I initially thought that nursing was my gift to the world. Ironically, it was only through my failure in nursing that I found my true calling: writing. But I am still proud to be a nurse.

The following chapters will follow a "story first, lesson second" format. Whenever you see ####, just pause and reflect. Think about the story I just told you for ten seconds, and then proceed to the lessons.

Walt Cummings, December 2017

Chapter 1: I Should Have Been A Doctor

"I hope I don't get fired," I whispered to myself.

The ancient doors to the Cardiac ICU moaned as I walked through.

"A big moan just for me," I whimpered.

I almost crapped my pants, much like the patient in room 1. I had just finished my ICU orientation in less than six weeks. I felt like a virgin floating to a new unit! The nurses were new, too, as were the smells emanating from the patient rooms. I was 24 years old on the night shift and still had no idea what I was doing. I had had a disastrous experience so far, but the hospital had such a deep need for nurses that they kept me on staff. The day had finally come; it was time for me to face the Cardiac ICU!

I received report and walked into a Japanese patient's room. Mr. Miyagi (you can't make this stuff up) was smiling and chatting with his wife. I was amazed by how a guy this healthy could be in an ICU.

"Piece of cake. I ain't getting fired today, baby!" I snickered to myself.

My patient in the other room looked pretty simple too. A patient on a ventilator with some bed sores. Tasty!

From 9pm to 11pm, I opened a conversation with a pretty Asian nurse and started to game her (this is what male nurses do on the night shift when there's nothing to do). She was quick to tell me that she had a boyfriend, so I proceeded to explain why her boyfriend was a loser. During my bashing, another nurse told me that Mr. Miyagi's vital signs were off.

"I'll be right back," I said with a wink.

As I walked into the room at 11pm, I saw that Mr. Miyagi was confused. There was a complete 180 degree difference from how he presented at 7pm.

"I don't feel so gooood," he belched.

My heart skipped a beat as I saw him open his mouth. He began to vomit purple blood. I grabbed the vomit bucket and started praying for the first time in my life.

"Please stop vomiting, Mr. Miyagi!" I screamed.

To my horror, Mr. Miyagi didn't stop puking. The room reeked of rotten sushi mixed with old blood. Purple vomit was rebounding off the bucket and falling on my face. I almost started to cry when I saw Mr. Miyagi's face turning blue. He was vomiting so much that he couldn't breathe! Mr. Miyagi was a geyser and I couldn't get him to stop.

As I tried to catch all the vomit, the charge nurse stepped in.

"Call a code!" she screamed to the nurse outside.

I started compressions as a team of people flooded the room. Every time I pounded on Mr. Miyagi's chest, bloody vomit would shower me. One nurse gave emergency medications as the respiratory therapist suctioned the patient's mouth. It was close to midnight, and my shift was just getting started.

Eventually, the Emergency doctor came in and took control of the Code Blue. Twenty more minutes dragged on as I took turns with the respiratory therapist giving chest compressions. People started to speculate where all the blood had come from. Perhaps he had been internally bleeding into his stomach for the last three days? Maybe his sutures had failed to hold up? The more people speculated, the more I wanted to shrink into the corner. I didn't know what hurt more: my wrists, or the fact that Mr. Miyagi had just been joking around with me at 7pm *that very shift*. Can you believe it was my wrists?

Forty minutes of compressions, defibrillations, and epinephrine injections came to a head as the healthcare workers gave up hope. The Emergency doctor officially called the time of death at 11:40pm. It was my first death, and I didn't know what to think. I was in shock. I still couldn't get over the fact that Mr. Miyagi was fully oriented just four hours earlier.

I held back tears as I dealt with the corpse. The charge nurse taught me how to pull away the lines and tubings from Mr. Miyagi's dead body.

"Stop shaking, please," she said. "You need to be more professional."

It was time to place the dead body into a bag. Once we finished the job, I called the family members to tell them their beloved Mr. Miyagi had just died in the middle of the night. An hour later, ten family members trudged into the room with tears in their eyes. Every fiber of my being wanted to cry with them, but I held myself together. I just hoped they didn't comment on the bloody vomit on my uniform.

I stuttered through my explanation of what had happened with Mr. Miyagi. I explained the accumulation of blood in his gut, the projectile vomiting that ensued, and the healthcare team's best attempts to save his life.

By the time the family members left, I was visibly shaken. It had been eight hours since I had eaten anything. I was also worried that the family would file a lawsuit, ending my career. I also couldn't get over the fact that I would probably get fired for negligence. It was at this point that the charge nurse told me that I would get a new admission from the Emergency Department. A second later, one of my fellow nurses told me my other patient had defecated and needed to be cleaned. I had no clue that so many things could hit me at once when everyone else was sleeping!

The rest of the night was a disaster. I made a critical mistake with the new admission's medications and had to work overtime. Did I mention that I didn't get to eat anything?

As I drove home at 8:30 am with vomit, urine, and feces on my uniform, there was only one thing running in my head: "I should have been a doctor."

####

Lesson One: **You will inevitably experience overwhelming shifts that will make you regret being a nurse**. I personally had these thoughts *every time* I drove back home from a shift. Dealing with death, CPR, blood, feces, urine, and family members is not easy and may be enough to cause people to quit their jobs. But the moment you tell yourself that you should have chosen another career, just remind yourself that the grass is not greener on the other side. What you are going through is difficult, but it is only temporary. All new nurses at the bedside pass through this phase, and it is completely normal to think negative thoughts. The reality is that every profession has its negatives. Even doctors have to go through grunt work. As a matter of fact, 60 percent of doctors would retire now if they could (access to the report can be found at: https://physiciansfoundation.org/research-insights/a-survey-of-americas-physicians-practice-patterns-and-perspectives/).

Action step: every time you think that you should have chosen another career, say the following out loud: "The grass is not greener on the other side. What I am going through right now is only temporary."

Lesson Two: When you get overwhelmed as a new grad (which will inevitably happen), ask for as much help as possible. I repeat: **liberally asking for help is the best thing you can do in the early stages.** For instance, when Mr. Miyagi was vomiting, I should have immediately called for help, rather than just trying to clean up the mess. Also, when I had to place Mr. Miyagi's corpse into a body bag, I had no idea what I was doing. The charge nurse had to step in because I was visibly struggling. I would have saved myself a lot of time if I had just asked for help earlier. To summarize lesson two: ask for help as if asking for help makes you look good (it actually does).

Action step: practice in front of a mirror, saying "I need your help" three times a day. When you actually do need help, it'll be easy to ask because you'll have practiced many times already.

Lesson Three: **Disasters happen when you get cocky.** Looking back, I could have been more prepared for Mr. Miyagi's condition if I had checked in on him at the top of every hour. At the very least, I would have seen his condition worsen. This would have likely spurred me to consult with another nurse just to make sure Mr. Miyagi was okay. Instead, what did I do? I tried to flirt with a girl and became distracted. Entire books can be written about Lesson Three, but I will only leave three guidelines on cockiness:

a) If you are on the night shift and think nothing will happen to your patients ("this is easy money!"), then you need to realize that countless patients have died because of that very mentality. If you catch yourself being cocky, just take one action: at the top of every hour, physically walk into your patients' rooms and ask how they are doing. Your physical assessment gives you a lot more information than a quick glance at vital signs.

b) If you are in your first six months of your nursing job, do not get lost in flirting with your female colleagues. You will inevitably come across this situation: the shift will appear to be easy, you will get bored, and then you'll feel an incredible urge to run the game on Sarah and Michelle, who are both single (and ready to mingle). When this situation happens, follow the advice from point a. That is, physically show up to your patients' rooms at least once every hour. You will inevitably flirt with your female colleagues, but don't get lost in the chatter.

c) Whenever you find yourself bored, ask yourself: what are the three worst things that can happen during this shift, and what can I do to prevent them? Are my rooms set up in such a way that I'll be prepared for these disasters?

Lesson Four: **Whenever you float to another unit, ask your coworkers if they know anything about your patients.** In Mr. Miyagi's case, I could have been more prepared if I had asked my fellow nurses if they knew anything about the patient's history. A good way to frame your question is: "do you have any advice for me for patient X?"

To sum up: Whenever you think that you should have chosen another career, remind yourself that the grass is not greener on the other side. Avoid stupidity by asking questions. Avoid cockiness by physically showing up to your patients' rooms every hour. Whenever you float, ask your new coworkers if they have any advice in the care of your patients.

Chapter 2: Why Am I Taking Orders From A Woman?

In your nursing career, you will run across women you despise. They will be impressively ugly and will remind you of men. You will even wonder if they have male body parts. Worst of all, these women will try to tell you what to do. You will get PISSED when this happens. The way you handle this anger will go a long way in your nursing career. Here's a story to highlight the lessons I've learned.

I first met Abbie on my third night in the ICU. If you had cut off her hair, she would have looked like Arnold Schwarzenegger (with smaller boobs). Her voice was as deep as his, too. She also must have eaten like Arnold because she reeked of eggs.

"I wonder if she has testicles?" I pondered when I first saw her.

"Hi Walt! It's so nice to meet you. I've heard really great things about you!" she said.

I appreciated her outgoing nature, but I knew that women who try too hard are usually compensating for something. I had met women like her before, and I wasn't impressed with the facade.

On Christmas Eve, I was working in an ICU bay with Abbie and Kaley, a travel nurse who didn't know the unit well. Things were going smoothly until the Emergency Department called to give report on Mr. Rice, a true mess. He was a 60 year old presenting with sepsis from a local nursing home. Nursing home workers are notorious for not giving a shit about their jobs. I wasn't surprised to find Mr. Rice with bed sores all over his buttocks, legs, and feet. His bed sores were full of pus and were at least half an inch deep. Two of his sores on his ass had maggots writhing in them.

"Oh my God!" screamed Kaley.

"Walt, be a man and take the maggots out!" yelled Abbie.

Annoyed, I grabbed a spoon and started scraping the larvae out.

"How dare this cunt delegate this to me. I will own her now!" I said to myself.

"Abbie, call the doc for admitting orders. Kaley and I will handle the wounds," I said.

Abbie wanted to be in control, so she fired back.

"No, patient safety has the first priority. We need to clean his body first," said Abbie.

"Abbie, this is *my* patient. I know what to do. Just do me a favor and call the doc for orders," I replied.

"No, you are a new grad. You're the one that needs to call the doc. Kaley and I will clean," she fired back.

The maggots started to jump with all the tension in the air. At this point, I was seriously ticked. Every fiber in my being wanted to call her a bitch and tell her to get out of my patient's room.

Rather than fight Abbie in front of Mr. Rice, I walked away and called the doc. Even though I wanted to win the argument, I knew the patient had the priority in this situation.

While I made the call, I could feel myself burning with anger. One more straw would break the camel's back.

The doctor ordered Propofol to sedate the patient. I asked one of the Respiratory Therapists to get it from the Pharmacy, at which point Abbie screamed:

"Walt! You can't do that! Therapists can't touch our medications!"

"SHUT YOUR TRAP, BITCH! This is my patient and you won't interfere anymore!" I yelled.

Abbie immediately broke into tears as Kaley tried to console her. The Respiratory Therapist ran away from the awkward situation. Mr. Rice continued to moan. Mr. Rice's maggots writhed in agony.

The rest of the night was interesting, because Abbie and I never exchanged another word. I had attacked her personality because I wanted to win. In doing so, I lost the respect of two coworkers.

####

Lesson One: **Swallow your ego.** Situations will occur where it will be you versus a female nurse. You will seriously resent one another. Eventually you two will have different opinions of how to care for a single patient, and you will try to tell each other what to do in an attempt to control the situation. However, the dispute will really be a matter of pride: who is going to win the argument? In such scenarios, **let go of your desire to win. Just do what is necessary for safe patient care, even if you have to lose an argument or look like a fool.** In my situation, I could have avoided humiliating Abbie if I had just suppressed my desire to win. That said, there are at least three obstacles for male nurses when fighting female nurses. First, you will feel offended that a female is telling you what to do. Second, you will think you are smarter than the female and will be less prone to listening to her. Third, your manly pride will want you to win the argument at all costs. All three factors make it very difficult for a male nurse to succumb to the demands of a female nurse, especially when the female nurse is not in a supervisory position over the male. It will hurt like hell to listen, but you should succumb if the demand makes sense and doesn't hurt the patient.

Action step: anytime a female colleague delegates something to you, just ask yourself: "Will this help my patient?" If so, then just do the task. If you really disagree with the delegation, then state your position and the reason. The worst case scenario is that you will have to ask help from another coworker.

Lesson Two: **Refrain from calling a female coworker a "bitch."** Seriously. Drop that word from you dictionary once you step onto the floor. Not only will that word probably get you fired, but you will regret using it. Remember: nursing is a small world. The ass you're kicking now will be the ass you will be licking in five years.

Action step: when you come across female colleagues that get under your skin, start telling yourself why you like such persons. For example, every time I saw Abbie, I could have told myself: "I like Abbie because she really cares about her patients." These self-statements would have made me resistant to calling Abbie a bitch, because my subconscious mind would have been conditioned to like her. If that doesn't float your boat, here is another action step: any time you're about to use the word "bitch," ask yourself if getting fired is worth the temporary feeling of victory that the word will give you.

Lesson Three: **Women communicate through "tending and befriending."** That is, they view work as an opportunity to nurture relationships. On the other hand, men work to exercise technical expertise and to advance in their careers. When talking with female coworkers, just realize that your interactions with them are not simply a means to exchange information. Your encounters with them significantly affect the way they feel. You have been warned!

Action step: when interacting with female nurses, tell yourself that "this woman wants to form a positive working relationship with me." This statement reminds you that women delegate tasks mainly because they seek control in chaotic situations, not because they want to hurt your pride. Men, on the other hand, are more prone to delegating tasks for the sake of showing people who's boss.

To sum up, let you go of your desire to win battles against female nurses. Don't use the B word. Realize that women are relational creatures. Interact with them not only to get the job done, but also to build rapport.

Chapter 3: How To Survive The Night Shift

"Can you work overtime?" asked the charge nurse Joe.
"How much?" I asked.
"Probably one or two hours. The day shift nurse will be late."
It was 5am, and I was working my fourth straight night shift. I was trembling from the lack of sleep and the sheer amount of coffee in my system. My body was screaming for shut eye, but the idea of getting paid at twice my hourly rate was too seductive. I was fantasizing about two hours of double time pay. My ego was salivating at the extra money, but my body begged for mercy. Guess who won?
"I can work extra," I said.
This is what you need to know about the night shift: not only does it suck physically, but it also drains you emotionally. It is completely unnatural to work from 7pm-7am and to sleep during the day time (if you can get any sleep, that is). Beginning on the third straight night shift, my hands start to shake. I become slow to respond, much like an 80 year old with dementia. I also become moody like a teenager on her period.
The fourth straight night shift is ten times worse. My entire body starts trembling like Michael J. Fox (sorry Mike), and I start hearing

things that no one else hears. Did I mention I'm taking care of patients the entire time?

Back to 5 am. After I agreed to overtime, I scrambled to the nursing lounge for my sixth cup of coffee. I was so dehydrated that my urine looked like dark orange juice. Also, I could no longer feel the Provigil (a cognitive enhancer) in my system, and I knew that caffeine's effects had plateaued. I would have to get through the next four hours like a zombie.

7 am rolled around, signifying the start of a new 12-hour shift. I started giving the morning meds. I was depending on muscle memory because I didn't have enough energy to think. I barely noticed the flood of the oncoming day shift nurses. A couple of them greeted me, but I just kept my mouth shut. After all, I couldn't tell the difference between real voices and the voices in my head. I didn't want anyone to think I was going crazy!

I started 8 am with another cup of coffee. As I stared at my computer screen pretending to chart, the pain in my shoulder escalated. It felt as if someone were jamming an ice pick down my right shoulder. The effects of decades of poor computer posture tend to strike on the night shift. The fact that I hadn't slept in 20 hours didn't help, either.

"Ohh Michelle, did you get your boob job?" I heard someone say. It sounded like one of the nurses to my right, but I couldn't tell the difference between her voice and the voice in my head.

9am came. I was so dizzy I couldn't walk in a straight line. I began to hate myself for loving money so much. To make matters worse, urine started to dribble out spontaneously. My farts were coming out uncontrollably, too. I didn't even care that my coworkers were scrambling away from me. I just wanted to stay alive!

10am rolled around, and I had no idea if the day shift nurse would come to relieve me. Walking was now painful. My arms felt as if they weighed fifty pounds, and my legs were as heavy as barbells. I could barely keep my eyes open. And even when they were wide open, the world was a blur. The worst part was that paranoia started settling in. Not only did I think my coworkers were conspiring against me, but I genuinely believed I was going to die. The catastrophic thoughts raced across my mind.

"The managers purposely made the day shift nurse come late to torture me!" said one voice.

"They're going to take my license away for malpractice!" screamed another.

"I can feel my heart beating out of my chest. Am I going to have a stroke?" said yet another.

I overheard some nurses expressing their concerns about me to the charge nurse.

"Is Walt okay? He looks like he's about to crash."

"He hasn't said anything to us all shift."

"His bay really smells."

It took me a minute to realize I was a danger to my patients. I needed to get out! I could feel my heart beating irregularly and was very close to just leaving the unit, not caring if I got fired.

At 10:15am, the charge nurse relieved me after seeing how I could barely keep my eyes open. The next 15 minutes were a blur as I trudged to my car. I brought some coke and a cup of coffee, even though I knew they wouldn't do anything. I had a feeling the drive home would be the most challenging task of my life.

I turned the radio all the way up to the most annoying music. Justin Bieber's "Baby" came at the right moment.

"BABY, BABY, BABY! It's time to live, baby!!" I screamed.

My self-induced adrenaline rush was enough to keep me awake until I got out of the parking structure. Once I hit the highway, I was literally drifting off every few minutes, oscillating between semi-asleep states and moments of sheer terror where others honked at me for veering off my lane. The coke, coffee, and max volume weren't enough.

Just to fight against my body shutting down, I started screaming and smiling like a psychopath. The surrounding cars increased their distance from me.

"When you're down to nothing, God has something!!" I yelled out loud.

I pretended I was a Pentecostal preacher and started dancing in my seat. I wondered when the police would start chasing me.

I was five minutes away from home and started laughing hysterically. I was acting, of course. Screaming and smiling were no longer stimulating enough to keep me awake. I now had to masturbate, laugh out loud, and yell obscenities to make it through the commute.

By the time I drove into my garage, I was amazed I was still alive. I collapsed onto my bed. As I drifted off to sleep, I asked myself if all that was worth 3.25 hours of double time pay.

"No, but at least I ejaculated," said the voice in my head.

####

Lesson One: **The only way to survive the night shift is to get 3-5 hours of sleep before your shift begins.** If you get more, you're lucky. Many nurses compensate for bad sleep by taking drugs or drinking ridiculous amounts of coffee. You can spot these nurses; they are usually obese, depressed, and oftentimes hairy. The point is that there are many artificial ways to battle against fatigue. But the only solution that works is consistent sleep. So how do you get quality sleep? In my experience, there are three ways. First, you need to set up a consistent schedule and stick to it. I personally would sleep in the same place at 9 am after every shift, allowing no deviations. Second, you need to sleep in a *completely dark* environment. I slept in my closet and placed towels in the crevices around the door to eliminate all sunlight. Third, you need to eliminate noise by using a white noise machine. The point is to trick your body into thinking it's night time.

In general, I don't recommend using sleeping pills or melatonin. Only use them if all other measures fail to get you enough sleep.

What do you do if you follow every trick in the book and still can't sleep? You only have two choices: either switch to the day shift or quit your job. Ultimately, your health and sanity have the first priority.

Lesson Two: **Never compromise your sleep just to make more money.** In other words, avoid working overtime on the night shift, even if you need the money. Remember the scene in *Gattaca* when the two adult brothers compete to see who can swim farther from the shore? The protagonist Vincent swims farther than his genetically superior brother because Vincent "never left anything for the swim back." *This advice is bullshit.* The reality is that at the end of every night shift, there's always the drive back home, the swim back to shore.

You need to leave some energy for this, or you could fall asleep at the wheel and die. Is it worth your life just to make some extra overtime cash?

Action step: whenever your charge nurse asks you to work overtime on the night shift, just say no. The drive back home is the most critical part of your night shift, because that's when you're the most prone to falling asleep.

Lesson Three: **If you're like me and you can barely tolerate the night shift, then schedule yourself to a maximum of two consecutive night shifts.** That is, avoid scheduling yourself to three or more straight night shifts. In general, people get their best sleep right before the first night shift. Every sleeping session after the first one tends to get worse. Because the quality of your sleep deteriorates with each consecutive night shift worked, you should minimize your exposure to strings of consecutive night shifts.

This is what the scenario looks like in real life: Assuming you get to self-schedule, your manager will give you a list with all the nurses on your unit and many boxes signifying nights you'd prefer to work. You will be tempted to just schedule yourself for three consecutive night shifts per week so you can have four straight days off. *Do not be seduced by how good this looks on paper.* Because each night shift takes a toll on your body, it's better to space your night shifts apart rather than work a bunch of them together. Please remember that working the night shift is a marathon, not a sprint. You need quality sleep, and working more than two consecutive night shifts kills your sleep.

Action step: Tell your manager that you can't work more than two consecutive night shifts due to health reasons. What do you have to lose? We're talking about your health here!

Lesson Four: **If you are close to falling asleep during your shift and have already maxed out on caffeine, then do not sit down.** We all go through these periods. The situation typically looks like this: you only get an hour of sleep (and oftentimes even less) before a shift, and you feel your body shutting down from 1 am onward. The key to surviving will be to stay active. Just stand up when charting and talk more with your coworkers. What I found especially helpful was doing jumping jacks and push ups in the restroom during breaks (seriously). The general rule of thumb is: your state will follow your physiology. So just get into peak state through movement, and energy will follow. Your alternative is to dump coffee down your throat, but you can only take so much caffeine.

Lesson Five: **Whenever you start falling asleep at the wheel, start jerking off and screaming.** I can honestly say that this strategy is the reason I am still alive today. I can't tell you how many times I've fallen asleep at the wheel, whether that be dozing off at a red light or sleeping on the highway going 65 miles per hour. *You need a way to change your state when full blast music, caffeine, and talking on the phone have failed.* Remember: the goal is to arouse yourself! That said, I have found that smiling, singing songs, and talking aloud to myself only work half the time. The only two strategies that have worked 100% of the time have been jerking off while screaming. Don't worry if you see cars increasing their distance from you. At least you will be awake!

To sum up the night shift chapter, you should aim for at least three hours of sleep before every shift. Avoid overtime. Avoid stretches of three or more straight shifts. Do not sit down if you feel your body is failing you. Jerk off and scream simultaneously at the wheel; it will keep you awake and make you feel good.

Chapter 4: I Want To Smash My Classmates

My dream was coming true: nursing school was about to start and I would be surrounded by beautiful women for the next four years. They would be young, dumb, and full of innocence. I was going to be a 19 year old cherry picker in a garden full of cherries! I had memorized the main strategies in The Game (by Neil Strauss) to get better at the art of Pick Up. "Seduce and Destroy!" became my mantra.

There was a slight issue, though. I had always been awkward around women. Every time I spoke with a pretty girl, I would start stuttering like a retard. To stop my lips from quivering, I'd bite down the inside of my lip and end up looking like a fish. But I decided to just step into the fire. Quivering or not, I was going in.

I was so amped before the first nursing meeting that I ran to the bathroom to relieve myself. Shameless, I walked into class with my chest out.

"You give praise, they give pussy!" I screamed to myself. I read that advice on a Pick Up forum and was committed to it.

I scanned the room like a drone. According to The Game, my chances of capture were highest with isolated women. Jackie sat in the corner with her breasts screaming "pick me, pick me!"

"You look a little lonely," I said.

"Oh shoot! Sorry, you scared me," said Jackie.

"Oh shoot!" I said, imitating her.

She chuckled. Things were looking good. Tony Robbin's strategy of body mirroring was working.

"I'm so glad you're funny. You're the first normal guy I've met in the last two weeks since coming to campus."

"I'm glad to meet you too; you're the first pretty girl I've seen on campus all week."

"You're a big liar! I'm Jackie by the way. It's nice to meet you."

"I'm Walt. By the way, something about you smells great."

"I'm a huge fan of Coco Chanel. Guess what flavor I'm wearing?"

"Your shoes look so nice. Where did you buy them?"

"Oh, I go to Macy's all the time."

"Me too. You've got a great taste for malls."

"Thanks so much! Should we sit a little closer to the back? People might think we're weird for sitting in the first row."

"I love the blouse you have on. It shows off your curves in just the right way."

"Aw, you're so sweet. I've been running a lot lately. I'm glad you noticed the results!"

I was running out of compliments.

"I gotta take a piss," I said.

As I scurried across the room, my heart fell into my stomach. How could I have botched such a great beginning?

"Recover, damnit. Recover now and change your state!" I yelped to myself. I stuck my chest back out.

When I returned, someone had taken my seat. Oh well. It was time to use my momentum on someone else. I scanned the room again for ladies in isolation. Blonde at nine o'clock!

"That's a nice backpack you have," I said.

"Thanks. Your backpack isn't so bad either," said Jenny.

"You haven't seen anything yet. Wait till you see my pencil box."

Jenny laughed. She looked like a typical blonde: skinny, tall, and busty. Just like the ones I fantasized about.

"I'm Jenny, by the way. You are?"

"I'm Walt, like Walter White."

"Why not Walt Disney?"

"Walt Disney only comes out to play on the weekend, so you're going to have to wait."

"Haha, I didn't know Indians were funny."

"There are many misconceptions about us. Did you know we also have big dicks?"

Jenny laughed again.

Playing the funny card seemed to be working. But how long could I sustain it? It was time for the "you give praise, she gives pussy" strategy.

"But seriously, though. That's a nice backpack you have there," I said.

"You really like this backpack, huh? I can sell it to you if you want."

"Your shirt looks nice too."

"Wow, thanks. You're a sweet talker, aren't you?"

"I like your mascara, Jenny."

"Umm, ok..."

"By the way, your curly hair looks great on you."

"Walt, I'm feeling a little uncomfortable."

My lips started quivering. There was a silence that lasted forever. I had messed up again! It was okay, though. I was feeling the flow and getting stimulated. I leveraged the momentum and wandered into the other corner to find the third cherry.

The girl next to me was Egyptian, an exotic beauty. My lips quivered a little more when I saw her push up bra. I continued to stare at the gems until the Egyptian introduced herself.

"Hi, my name is Abby."

"Oh, hi! I'm Walt. I was looking at your notes. You have some really good notes there."

"Oh really? I got these notes from a friend just the other week. They're new."

"I can tell."

"Want to grab them?"

"Sure!"

I reached for the papers on her desk. We both started laughing.

"I'm sorry, that was so rude of me to be staring at you like that," I said.

"That's okay. I dressed this way for a reason. I just broke up with my boyfriend, so the attention makes me feel better."

"I feel better too."

"I don't mean to be rude, but I didn't know people like you went into nursing. What's an Indian guy like you doing here?"

"Scanning for good notes."

We had immediate chemistry. Three years later, we went to a bar and hooked up.

####

Let's get one thing straight: I advocate pursuing your female classmates not for the sexual enjoyment, but for the lessons you learn. Bodily enjoyment is temporary, but the lessons of your pursuit will pay dividends decades from now. Obviously, your priority in school should be to get good grades and test scores. But it is inevitable you will chase women in your class. Follow my advice only if you have your grades handled and have free time. Eventually, you will grow to view women as more than pieces of meat. Until you grow to that point, you should just try your best to have fun and learn.

On to the real talk. It's been several years since I graduated from nursing school. Guess how many of my classmates I keep in touch with? Zero. This means that you have nothing to lose. Your mindset should be to have fun and to take advantage of this precious time in nursing school. When you're 40 years old, you'll realize that nursing school is a unique opportunity. Never again will you be surrounded by so many young, beautiful women.

Lesson One: **Persevere. You will fall on your face many, many times.** How do you persevere when you feel like the only guy in the room? I recommend using the **three-step momentum theory** from my story above. Before class begins, make it your goal to talk with three girls. It doesn't matter if the girl is ugly or if you don't like her. You just need to get started! Once you initiate conversation with the first girl, the interaction will naturally end. Start a conversation with another girl. Then go on to the next one. As you go from conversation to conversation, you will build momentum. By the time you reach the third and fourth girls, you will be "in state" and feeling the flow. Conversation will roll off your tongue and your confidence will be sky high. Just remember *to have fun and to not care about the outcome*. Use this strategy before and after class because these down times are when relationships are built.

Use the three-step momentum theory until you've talked with all the girls in your class. You will eventually talk to every girl, and your gut will tell you which ones you have a shot with. Once you've talked with each girl, start focusing on the ones with whom you have chemistry. In general, you will click with 10% of the girls you approach. This means that 90% of the girls won't be interested.

Lesson Two: **Once you have found the girls you have chemistry with, keep it cool for at least one year. Make your move only after they are comfortable with you.** Let's say you're in a class of 60 people. You will naturally click with at least 10% of them (the *sexy six*). Upon identification, *do not* be aggressive. That is, don't ask the members of the *sexy six* out on dates, don't invite them to drink, and don't make moves on them in general for at least one year. If you make moves aggressively, they will know immediately you're trying to get into their pants. I recommend spending the first year nonchalantly. Only talk with members of the *sexy six* in unforced, natural environments. Once a certain feeling of naturalness, openness, and spontaneity is secured, you can make your move. That said, the one year time frame is not set in stone. The process may only take six months. The take home message is that it will take time for the feeling of spontaneity to happen. Let it develop without trying to force anything. Then, you can pounce.

Occasionally, you'll meet a girl in nursing class who is completely open. That is, she is down *right now*. In such cases, just take immediate action. Remember that your females classmates are in their early 20s and will never be more horny in their lifetimes (the same is true for you).

Lesson Three: **Ignore the fact that they have boyfriends. These relationships will dissolve over time.** You should expect that 90% of your female classmates will be in relationships. Be encouraged! From the ages of 18-22, these relationships are temporary. Practically speaking, this means that you should talk to a girl even if she has a boyfriend. That these young women think they will get married to their boyfriends is a joke.

Lesson Four: **Procrastination is your biggest enemy.** In our nursing class, we had a huge yacht party right before graduation. It had a dance floor, an open bar, and food. In other words, it was a perfect environment for people to show their true colors. I was amazed as I saw guys finally making their moves on the girls they wanted! After four years of inaction, these guys thought they could capture at the very end on a drunken boat party. They were wrong! Try your best to learn from these losers. You should be making moves (going to parties, drinking, going rock climbing, etc.) throughout your four years, especially after your first year of playing it cool. Remember: consistent action is key. Don't wait until your final yacht party to make a move!

Lesson Five: **Don't waste your time with the one liners and magic tricks that Pick Up Artists use. All you need is confidence.** But what if you don't have confidence? The answer is that you have to *act as if you have confidence*. You become whoever you pretend to be. See Lesson One for how to build momentum when you feel no confidence.

Your chances of getting laid will be very high if you follow my advice. The funny thing is that when you do get laid, you will probably feel empty. The real gem is realizing the only things that matter are consistency of action and perseverance over time. You will learn that success requires action, even though you don't feel like doing anything.

To sum up, persevere. Once you've identified the girls you have chemistry with, wait one year until making a move. Don't let relationships stop you. Just get started! Confidence will be your biggest friend, not little tricks.

Chapter 5: I Want To Be A CRNA

"Wow, that's a small hole," I thought.

It was my second month of clinicals in CRNA school. I was looking at the back of the patient's mouth to see how hard it'd be to intubate, which is the practice of putting tubes down people's airways to help them breathe. At this point I was obsessed with intubations, much like a teenage boy is obsessed with porn. The feeling of putting a tube down someone's airway was orgasmic. In fact, the glottic opening to the airway looks like a second vagina. It is small, wet, and usually wide open. Putting a tube through the hole was the mental equivalent of penetration, and my ego wanted more of it.

Walking to the OR, I realized the intubation would be too tough with a standard approach. I needed a special tool called the glidescope.

Eventually, the patient was wheeled into the OR. I put on the monitors as the anesthesiologist gave the sleeping drugs. It was time to penetrate!

I placed the glidescope into the patient's mouth, looking at the live-monitor to make sure I was in the right place. Once I was deep enough, I saw the glottic opening.

"Rape me!" I imagined the glottic opening saying.

I smiled. Then, I grabbed the endotracheal tube and tried to slide it down, following the natural curvature of the glidescope. For some reason, I couldn't advance the tube further than a couple of inches. There seemed to be a blockage.

"Keep your eye on the mouth, not the monitor," said the CRNA.

"Don't be too forceful," said the anesthesiologist.

I had two choices: remain quiet or ask for help. I decided to keep my mouth shut. After all, I could still see the glottic opening on the monitor.

After my fourth attempt to insert the tube, I was frustrated. I rammed the tube one last time with anger, creating a gaping hole in the soft palate.

"Oh shit," I said.

"Ok, move out. It's my turn," said the CRNA.

My heart sank as I saw the mouth fill up with blood. I grabbed the yankeur to suction the fluids out. The CRNA had a tough time, too. The tube just wouldn't advance. Maybe the cause was that the tube kept going into the big-ass hole I had just created?

We took a pause and ventilated the patient. The tension was thick; no one knew why the patient was bleeding so much, except for me. We called in the male anesthesiologist because the female anesthesiologist in the room had Parkinson's disease and was useless. She couldn't even wipe her own ass!

While the CRNA ventilated the patient, I grabbed another device called the C-MAC, the glidescope's cousin. The C-MAC had a thin, flexible cable whose movements could be controlled (think of the movements a worm can make; that's the C-MAC). The CRNA grabbed the C-MAC and guided the cable into the patient's mouth while I gave the patient some IV steroids to stop the inflammation.

At this point, the obese male anesthesiologist waddled into the room.

"Extend your left arm and go in slower," he barked.

"Keep your back straight and stop shaking," chimed Mrs. Parkinson's.

My CRNA handled the pressure like a pro. Once the cable reached the glottic opening, we slid the endotracheal tube down along the cable until the tube went into the airway. It took 30 minutes to intubate the patient!

I stopped hyperventilating as I realized the patient was going to live. The bleeding had decreased significantly, and we were proceeding through the case as if nothing had happened. To cover my ass, the CRNA called in an oral surgeon to check out the source of bleeding. Once he arrived, I started praising God. A guy to fix the hole I created!

"I've never seen a hole that big in someone's mouth," said the oral surgeon.

"I'm a beginner, sorry. Will it cause permanent damage?" I asked.

"Nah, I'll just stitch it up and it should completely heal in less than a month."

"Give me one second. I want to take a picture of the hole," said the CRNA.

"Yes, me too!" said the anesthesiologist with Parkinson's.

To my horror, the anesthesia providers whipped out their phones and took pictures.

"Wait, isn't this against the law?" I asked.

"Be quiet and chart, kid," said Mrs. Parkinson's.

When the case was done, I went into the staff lounge and found my CRNA showing her coworkers the gaping hole!

"Look at what my student did today," said my CRNA.

"You can't be serious," said a coworker.

"I've never seen anything like it. The intubation took 30 minutes and we needed both anesthesiologists in the room. We had to call in an oral surgeon to close the hole! The entire case lasted more than six hours," said my CRNA.

All I wanted to do was tell her to shut up. But if I did, she'd probably be provoked to tell my director. Little did I know that she had already texted the director within an hour of the hole creation.

As I walked out of the hospital that night, my heart sank again. The news had spread like wildfire, and my classmates were well aware of my mishap as the "mouth raper." I knew that if the students knew, then the director would inevitably find out, too.

One month later, I withdrew from CRNA school. Analyzing my own actions, I realized that I watched the clock like a hawk during clinical hours, indicating that I didn't like my role. I also shied away from IV insertions like a pussy. I also asked a CRNA one time if I could leave at 3pm so I could finish care plans for the next day, showing a lack of interest in the actual work of anesthesia. All these actions showed a lack of passion on my part. All in all, it was a good career decision to withdraw.

####

l am not here to bash the CRNA field. I think it's a great career choice if you want to make good money. That said, these are points I wish someone would have told me before I tried to become a CRNA.

Lesson One: You will be the Nurse Practitioner (NP) in the anesthesia world. In the story above, my CRNA did the grunt work, dealing with my mistake while the anesthesiologists stood there barking orders. Guess who took credit for the case? You guessed right! It was the anesthesiologist with Parkinson's. Even though my CRNA was the hero, she was still just a mid-level provider.

When I was 18 years old, I thought that giving anesthesia would bring a certain loftiness to my life. That is, giving anesthesia would make me a big time nurse, some kind of quasi-doctor. The reality is that as a CRNA, you will be viewed as a nurse and nothing more. Just as doctors view Nurse Practitioners as unequal mid-level providers, anesthesiologists and surgeons view CRNAs as second-rate providers. As a CRNA once told me, "you are the surgeon's bitch." Beg to differ? Then shadow a CRNA and observe how he/she interacts with the surgeon. More likely than not, you'll see that CRNAs stroke their surgeons. CRNAs change their communication styles when talking with surgeons, much like daughters change their communication styles when talking with their fathers.

Action step: ask yourself if you are okay with being a Nurse Practitioner. For all intents and purposes, you will be the NP of anesthesia.

Lesson Two: You won't be the captain of the ship. You won't be second in command, either. Here's the pecking order: the surgeon is at the top, the anesthesiologist is second in command, and the CRNA is the third wheel. That is, the CRNA does the work, and the credit goes to the MDs.

Action step: visualize yourself asking a doctor to do things. Visualize yourself needing permission to do what you think is right for a patient. If you are okay with this, then being a CRNA may be right for you.

Lesson Three: **You will be making $160,270 per year, which is the median salary of CRNAs in 2016 (https://www.bls.gov/oes/current/oes291151.htm).** Half will make less and half will make more. For nine years I fantasized about bringing in $200,000-$300,000 per year while sitting on a stool and playing poker on my iPad. I never considered the actual salary statistics. If you're committed to making more than $200,000, you will likely need to practice in a rural area or work multiple jobs. Or you might need to get into ownership. The point is that half of CRNAs make less than $160,270. To make more than the median salary, you're going to have to do more than sit on a stool and play poker in one hospital.

Action step: repeat the following phrase: "I understand that if I want to make more than $200,000 as a CRNA, I will likely have to work overtime hours, work more than one job, work in a rural area, or get into ownership."

Lesson Four: **The DNP requirement does not uplift the face of nurse anesthesia. It actually makes the field less attractive to aspiring nurses.** If schools are moving toward the doctoral requirement for entry-level practice as a CRNA, then it begs the question: why don't students just become doctors instead? Let's look at this from an 18 year old's viewpoint (this analysis will be oversimplified for the sake of argument).

Becoming a CRNA will require four years getting an undergraduate degree, one to two years getting ICU experience, and four years getting a doctoral degree in nurse anesthesia. That's 9-10 years to become a "nurse anesthesia doctor." What if the 18 year old wanted to be a traditional doctor? That would require four years getting an undergraduate degree, four years getting a medical degree, and three to four years of residency. That's 11-12 years to become a "doctor." Both the CRNA route and the MD route will generally take a decade to complete, with the MD route being marginally longer. If this is the case, why would a young man pursue a CRNA career over an MD career? He is better off trying to be a traditional doctor with no limitations on practice rather than a nurse-doctor whose role is limited and requires supervision in many cases.

Action step: read the following sentence and answer from your heart. "An anesthesiologist makes more money than a CRNA and has fewer limits on his practice. A CRNA makes less money than an anesthesiologist and has more limits on his practice. Both routes take around a decade to finish, with the MD route being longer. Which route makes more sense?"

Lesson Five: **Being a CRNA is 99% boredom and 1% sheer terror.** When the shit hits the fan in anesthesia, all hell breaks loose. Emergencies usually happen in the beginning when providers are securing the airway, or at the end when the providers are wakening the patient. That said, being a CRNA is similar to being a pilot. Crashes usually happen on take-off and landing, not when the plane is in cruise control. The vast majority of the time, the pilot is going through the motions and enjoying the auto-pilot part of his job. In the same vein, the CRNA goes on autopilot while the surgeon is operating. The stessors for the CRNA mainly occur at the beginning and end of the operation. All that said, I wish I had known that the role of the CRNA is not intellectually stimulating. You make your money off your ability to handle the extremes at the 1%. The name of the game is living with the boredom and making it through the emergencies.

Action step: write down (yes, grab a pen and start jotting) what your dream job looks like. How do you feel in this job, and what are you doing? Now look at your writing. Does your dream job include being bored 99% of the time? If so, being a CRNA might be right for you.

Lesson Six: **Only be a CRNA if you have a passion for it**. How do you know if you have a passion? You will have to read your own actions. Do you read anesthesia books in your spare time? Do you memorize and read up on drugs as a hobby? Do you read about and practice intubations, even though you're not in school? Examine your actions to see if you actually have a passion for being a CRNA, and go from there.

Action step: ask yourself the following question: "do I study anesthesia in my free time?" If you don't, then you probably aren't passionate about anesthesia.

To sum up, being a CRNA is being the Nurse Practitioner of the anesthesia world. You won't be in command. You will be making close to $160,270 a year, not $300,000. The DNP may not be worth it. The job is 99% cruise control and 1% terror. Be passionate if you're going to pursue the career!

Chapter 6: Disciplinary Action And Getting Fired

Job#1

My first nursing job was in a rehab unit, which looked like a nursing home in the 1950s. I basically had to give pills and wipe people's asses after they had strokes and spinal injuries. When I was 24, I was passionate about keeping my back straight to avoid back pain. The nursing gods had a sense of humor, because I was constantly straining my back by moving and pulling on obese men.

In my second month I was assigned to Luis, a 5'6," 260 pound fat fuck. No one was surprised when he suffered a massive stroke, which left him semi-paralyzed on his left side. After seeing the CT scans, I was surprised he could even move. I went into Luis' room and found a bunch of family members.

"Good morning Luis! How are you?" I asked.

"Puto," he responded.

"Sorry, he can barely speak. The stroke must have affected his language center," said his daughter Jessica, who was no more than 16 years old.

"Thank you. Luis, I'm Walt and I will be your nurse today."

"Puto, puto," said Luis.

Jessica and her teenage boyfriend started laughing.

"Luis is calling you a little bitch!" said Jose, the boyfriend. The entire family erupted in laughter.

"I'll make you wipe his ass, beaner," I muttered under my breath.

"Sorry, that seems to be his favorite word today," said Jessica. "He'll start moaning when he needs to go the restroom."

Like clockwork, Luis started moaning. It sounded like someone was fingering him.

"Time for the nurse to do his job," said Jose.

I fought my urge to talk back. I asked the family members to leave, requesting that Jessica and Jose stay in case I needed help.

"Why do we have to stay? It's your job to help him go to the bathroom," said Jose with a smirk.

"Luis is a big guy and I might need help moving him," I responded.

"Mmm! Mmmmm!" moaned Luis. Green diarrhea seeped from his semen-stained whitey tighties.

Jessica grabbed a wheelchair as Jose and I secured Luis in a sitting position. I applied a gait belt around Luis' waist, locked his knees between mine, and used Luis' right leg as a pivot to swing him into the chair. Jessica wheeled the massive man into the restroom, where I used the pivot strategy to get him onto the toilet.

"Wow, that's pretty good for a nurse. I'm not sure if you need me," said Jose.

"I'll need you when Luis is done taking care of business," I quickly replied.

Luis started raping the toilet. The diarrhea splashes were louder than his grunts! I blocked the main door so Jessica and Jose couldn't leave, and we didn't say a word for ten minutes as I let the smell of shit fill the room. Jessica and Jose were shaking in horror as Luis started moaning louder. Obviously, they had never seen a grown man with diarrhea unleash himself. When he was done, Luis closed his eyes and stuck his tongue out in pure exhaustion.

"Jessica, I need you to hold the wheelchair steady. I will help Luis stand, and Jose will clean him up," I said.

"Nah, fuck you. I ain't wiping his ass," said Jose.

"It's either you or your girlfriend, because neither of you is strong enough to lift Luis."

"I'll do it," said Jessica.

"You're going to just give up and let your girlfriend wipe her dad's ass?" I asked Jose.

"Yea, she can do it. I'll hold the wheelchair," he replied.

"What a little bitch," I said to myself. Deep inside, I was delighted they were listening to me. It was unconventional for me to delegate duties to family members.

I locked Luis' knees between mine, and I lifted him off the toilet like a powerlifter. Jessica squealed and wiped Luis' ass cheeks, avoiding the golden anus.

"Take care of the butthole," I directed.

"Don't talk to my girlfriend like that," shot Jose.

I smirked.

Luis moaned some more as his teenage daughter rubbed the shit from his asshole. When the diarrhea was wiped away, I moved Luis onto the wheelchair. At this point, Jessica broke out in tears.

"I can't believe you made me do that," she cried.

"This is your dad, not mine!" yelled Jose.

"This is how our relationship works, huh? You say you love me, and then I have to do the dirty work. Why can't you just stand up for me?"

"So it's my fault that you volunteered to clean your dad?"

"Only because you were too scared to!"

"It's the nurse's fault for making us do his job!"

"What's wrong with helping Luis out?" I interrupted with feigned concern. "It should be an absolute joy to help family members."

Jessica and Jose continued to fight, so I told them to get out of the room. Right when Jose reached the hallway, I grabbed his arm.

"Who's the puto, now?" I asked.

"I'm reporting you to your director," he screamed.

"I didn't break any laws, beaner," I said.

Barely three days passed before I was called into my manager's office. Not surprisingly, she scolded me for delegating my job to family members. Because I didn't break any laws, I walked away with a slap on my wrist. From that point onward, I began to act more aggressively because I was confident I could get away with things.

My delegation of duties to family members slowly evolved into other kinds of mischief. By the time the third month rolled around, I started fabricating patient's blood pressures. In my mind, it was justified because in the rehab unit there were no automatic blood pressure machines. That is, the nurses had to take blood pressure measurements the old fashioned way with stethoscopes. Imagine having to do that for five different patients! The process took forever and I had no patience. Besides, the doctors and physical therapists didn't look at the vital signs, anyway. Needless to say, I was quick to justify all my actions, however blatantly wrong they were.

My time in the rehab unit came to a head when I missed an order for heparin. From that point, I was placed under a gigantic microscope. The charge nurses inspected my charting as if I didn't know English. They reported that I didn't scan medications, that I left medications in patients' rooms unattended, and that I handled sharps carelessly. It didn't help that I "networked" with other managers in the hospital to escape from the unit. Of course, word got back to my manager, who saw a picture of a young man taking shortcuts and making his getaway. Not surprisingly, I was suspended so management could gather evidence. Two days later I was called into the Human Resources office, where my manager was sitting next to Donna, the VP of Human Resources.

"How are you, Walt?" asked Donna.

"Good, how did the investigation go?" I answered. My heart was racing.

"It was great. Your manager and I were sharing stories of our dogs and how they're both having little puppies."

"It's as if our own families are being extended," chimed my manager.

"Let's cut the crap, ladies. I want to know the outcome of the investigation."

There was a pause. My manager changed her tone and filled me in.

"Walt, we have never had to deal with a new grad in this way before. You've been with us for less than six months, and many issues have arisen just in the last four weeks. First, you falsified documentation, saying that you gave an antibiotic even though the patient was not in the unit. Second, you failed to give heparin to a patient, even though the doctor told you he was inputting a heparin order. Instead of asking the charge nurse how to give it, you didn't say anything and waited for us to catch the mistake. The charge nurses have also reported grave concerns about patient safety. Not only do you leave sharps in patient rooms, but you also leave narcotic pills unattended. No prudent nurse would conduct him or herself in the way you have acted."

"Everyone makes mistakes. I'm asking for another chance," I said.

"Let me finish, please. There have been serious concerns with you delegating your work to family members. We also know that you've been talking with other managers, even though we have spent over $60,000 on your new grad training. Due to your negligence and gross misconduct, we have decided to terminate your employment with this hospital effective immediately."

I stared in disbelief. How could they be so merciless with a new grad?

"I don't know what to say," I muttered.

"The security guard will guide you outside. Please take all your possessions from your locker, return your badge, and leave the building," said Donna.

As the guard escorted me out from the HR building and into the rehab unit, I sensed a dramatic shift. The nurses looked at the ground, refusing to give me eye contact. When I entered the nursing lounge, two nurses left without saying a word. A deep sense of paranoia settled in. I got fired and no one wanted to talk with me! Was my career over in just six months? It would be next to impossible to find another job with such little experience.

That night of my first firing was interesting. I cried like a little bitch until the sun came up.

Job#2

It took two months for me to find another nursing job. This time, I was going to be trained as a new grad in the ICU on the night shift.

The new hospital was in the middle of the ghetto, serving mostly fat and poor people. It was going to be a churn and burn environment!

I made it through five months on the night shift before trouble came around the corner. Apparently, word had spread that I was a crazy dude. Again, I was suspended for a couple of shifts before I had to meet with the VP of Human Resources, Dorris. She was a woman suffering from the triple threat: she was black, female, and old. Naturally, she was loud and sassy to compensate.

"Walt, my nurses have been submitting some unique complaints about you. It's been reported that you show up super early to work, and that you roam the hospital."

"I show up early because I'm on the night shift and have to beat traffic. If I left my house at 6pm for a 7pm start, it'd take two hours to get here," I said.

"Why are you roaming the hospital?"

"I'm not. I'm simply headed to the computers to check my email."

"You need to be checking your email on your own time, not company time. Walt, I need you to be honest. The charge nurses on the fifth floor have reported that you showed up last week at 5pm to the Direct Observation Unit. But you don't even work there! Why are you going to a unit so early where you don't work?"

"Well, I regularly float to the DOU from the ICU, so I feel that the DOU is my second base. Also, they don't serve coffee in the ICU, so I just get it from the DOU."

It looked like my cheapness in refusing to buy coffee was being interpreted as intrusion.

"You need to stick to your unit, buddy. Another thing concerns me: when a charge nurse from the DOU asked you what you were doing there so early, she reported that you said 'I like the eye candy.'"

Suddenly it hit me; some of the female nurses thought I was a pervert trying to check on them while they were working!

"Wow, this is a complete misunderstanding," I said. "I literally told the charge nurse that I liked the candy. I was specifically referring to the candy in the jar in the charge nurse room that's offered to every nurse on the floor. I am in no way trying to hit on the female nurses."

"So you were specifically referring to the candy?"

"Yes, the candy is free. Look, the only reason I show up early is that I want to avoid traffic going west on the freeway. My behavior has nothing to do with eye candy!"

"Explain something else to me, Walt. Some DOU nurses filed a complaint the other day, saying you left your shift in the ICU at midnight last friday and wandered into the DOU. They said you stayed in the unit for seven hours, drinking coffee and taking one of the computers. You weren't on staff on the DOU, though!"

"The reason I went to the DOU for seven hours was that I had an appointment to see the director of the Cardiac ICU at 7:30am that morning. I had to keep myself awake in front of a computer until the meeting so I could get some sleep later on. I didn't interact with any of the nurses, nor did I get in anyone's way."

I wasn't bullshitting. Everything I said was true. But Dorris continued to stare at me like I was a psychopath. In her mind, I was a coffee loving rapist that liked to show up early to roam the halls for fresh meat. All I truly wanted to do was avoid heavy traffic and get some coffee before my shift started!

"Look," I continued. "There's a simple solution. I just won't show up to the DOU anymore. I will only drink the coffee there when I am designated to float."

"Walt, I'm just getting started. People from the ICU have been complaining, too. They have said that you eat yogurt in the bathroom and leave big messes in the restroom. They also say you are odd with patients, you lunge at doors, and that you have abnormally wide stances when charting. Do you have a psychiatric history I should know about?"

I almost laughed out loud. I ate yogurt and drank coffee to help me take massive shits at 6pm. My usual target was the staff bathroom near the front entrance to the ICU. My shit was so ferocious that I clogged the ICU toilet a couple of times. Did I mention that the smells were less than aromatic? As for being odd with patients, I was curious to see what the specific allegations were. The body posture complaints were icing on the cake. I was just trying to keep my back straight!

"Okay, I get it," I said. "I have some idiosyncrasies. But nothing you've mentioned so far has anything to do with my job performance. I want to be clear: I don't have any kind of psychopathology."

"If my nurses have serious concerns about your psychological health, that makes me very concerned, too."

"I bet I'm clearer in the head than most nurses here."

"I need all this strange behavior to stop. The worst case is that the patients start complaining about you. Things haven't gotten to that point, but I'm warning you that things may be going that route if you continue your act."

"Dorris, I'll stop showing up so early. But I'll tell you this: I will keep eating candy, I will keep eating yogurt and coffee in the bathroom, and I will continue to keep my back straight. Nothing you have said has anything to do with patient safety. That being said, you have no grounds to take disciplinary action. Now if you'll excuse me, I have to take a shit."

I stood up, farted in her face, and left the room. I headed straight to my favorite bathroom in the ICU and unleashed myself for the last time. As I released the yogurt and coffee in my system, I laughed at the glorious smells emanating from my asshole. I left the bathroom without flushing the toilet. I then went up to the DOU, grabbed some candy, and took one last sip of the fresh coffee (did I mention it was free)?

I didn't care that she was the VP of Human Resources. I was completely jaded and needed to move on. The fact was that the director of the Cardiac ICU wouldn't let me transfer to his unit. Plus, I was fed up with pushing, pulling, and wiping 300 pound patients addicted to fried chicken. I ended up resigning before they could fire me.

Job#3

When I started my new ICU nursing job (which was my third job in one year), I was pretty excited. Although it was in the ghetto, the medical center was the newest hospital in New York. The patient rooms had HD television sets, patient beds worth more than $20,000, and the newest medication pumps. More importantly, the hospital had state of the art Keurig coffee machines I could abuse all day. The only downside was that everyone was uptight. I was convinced that if you tried to hammer a needle up anyone's asshole, you'd fail miserably. The fact of the matter was that the hospital was re-opening after the old hospital had shut down for ten years, and we didn't know how things would work out. The old hospital was renowned for being unsafe and giving substandard care. In fact, at the nadir of the old hospital's existence, a nationally televised segment showcased footage of a man dying in the Emergency Department from a heart attack. The only person that made contact with the man was a janitor, who starred at the man writhing in pain and subsequently walked away. It was no wonder the old hospital was known as Satan's hole.

I had been hired two months before the hospital was to reopen its doors. During lunch, I would wander next door to the urgent care center. I had heard that doctors from the old hospital were now working there, treating patients with minor health conditions and killing time before retirement. I wanted to hear bloody stories. Countless people had told me Satan's hole was bad. How big and bad was the hole?

On a sunny afternoon, I walked into the urgent care center and went straight to the staff lounge to poke around. A chubby black man in his fifties waddled into the room.

"Hey Salan, how are you?" I asked, reading his name badge.

"I'm doing well. I'm guessing you're an employee from next door?"

"Yes, and I want to be in the best position to help the new hospital. Can you give me an idea of what the old hospital was like?"

"That depends. Do you like gunshot wounds?"

"I dream about them every night. I also like strokes, heart attacks, and cancer."

"You know, you've got balls coming to this building. No one from the new hospital ever comes here."

"What can I say? I have a fascination with Satan's hole."

"All I have to say is that you better enjoy the calm before the storm. Back in the day, we'd have patients with gunshot wounds coming in almost every night. We're talking about young men in their twenties coming in at 3 am, bleeding and sometimes crying for their mamas. There was one night where three gunshot patients came through the door. I got a taste of hell."

"What happens when those patients come in through the doors?"

"It depends on where they get shot. Some of them come in dead, others come in the late stages of shock. They don't die from the bullet; they die from blood loss, infection, or sepsis."

"Is that the craziest thing that happens?"

"Almost. You'll see all kinds of things at night. You'll witness stab wounds from domestic violence, rape wounds, attempted suicides gone wrong, and much more. Night time is when the monkeys come out to play."

"I heard that doctors and nurses would get robbed when they tried to get to their cars."

"That happened only to the employees who went out alone. Just stay in groups and you'll be fine. Also, I'd recommend bringing a shitty car to work and parking next to expensive cars. Keep your possessions safe."

"Kinda like parking my crappy bike next to a fancy one so the thief won't target mine?"

"Exactly. I think you'll be in good shape. If anything, you'll learn more about yourself, including how you handle stress and conflict. More importantly, you'll learn how to handle lies from the media. You see, we gave great care in the old hospital. We shed blood, sweat, and tears for all our trauma patients. But the media only gave you the negative side of the story. Not once did they highlight the lives we saved."

"What's the best advice you have?"

"Maintain your sense of humor. When you feel like quitting, remember you're in Satan's hole."

Salan walked out with a smile. I left the urgent care center with a renewed sense of purpose. *Gunshot wounds*, for crying out loud! I was about to see what I was made of.

When the hospital doors opened, I was underwhelmed. Because we were under the microscope, the administrators regulated the patient flow. Outside hospitals sent us relatively healthy patients just so we could have a census and "look good." Practically speaking, there were times when the ICU had no patients at all, so I would have nothing to do for 12 hours.

At 12am, I'd get to know my coworkers really well. Some respiratory therapists would try to hide in the equipment room and catch a couple of hours of sleep. Other nurses would lie down in patient rooms and watch porn on their phones. Yet others would gossip all night, talking trash about their husbands, past relationships, and phobias. I learned a great deal about my coworkers and realized that most of them were downright *crazy*.

Perhaps the greatest lesson was this: being bored out of your mind for 12 hours is unhealthy, especially in the middle of the night. At 3 am, I would jack myself up with coffee and start writing emails to myself. I wrote about my fantasies, the coworkers I hated, and what I would do to them if God didn't exist (I told you it's unhealthy to be *that* bored). Weirdly enough, I was having fun. It was great to fantasize about hurting my enemies while getting paid! Unfortunately, I didn't know that all my emails were being scrutinized. Even though I only drafted emails and never sent them, the security personnel read everything I had to say about my coworkers.

One night, I came in excited to work because we had no patients. I had great fantasies to journal about! As usual, I walked into a conference room as a shortcut to get to the restroom to take my nightly shit. I ran into my director, a security guard, and the VP of Human Resources, who were plotting on how to intercept me. I had walked into a trap!

"How could I have fucked up again? We don't even have any patients!" I screamed to myself.

"Walt, we were just looking for you!" said my director.

"Perfect timing! Go ahead and have a seat," said the VP.

"Obviously, I did something wrong if the security guard is here," I said.

The VP sighed loudly, stared at me, and shook her head. She had been working for twelve hours and now head to deal with me.

"Walt, I have some questions for you. The director of security forwarded me some emails. 'Fuck these niggers. I wonder how many of them will die in this shithole?' Does this sound familiar to you?"

"The word nigger is a term in my native tongue," I said. I was panicking inside. If they had read that draft, then they surely would have caught the others.

"What about this: 'Fuck Liz. I will slit that bitch's throat and ram a jackhammer up her pussy. Fuck her and her entire family. The throat will be the second vagina as I slit it and see how much blood pours out.' Which Liz are you referring to?"

I was actually referring to my charge nurse, who I thought was a dumbass. Unfortunately for me, the CEO of the hospital was also named Liz.

"I wasn't referring to the CEO," I muttered.

"How about this: 'These bitch ass charge nurses think they can tell me what to do? Fucking over-the-hill cunts who can't even eat right. Go home and have more kids, bitches.'

"Walt, do you have a psychiatric history? We have read all these emails and are concerned you are plotting to hurt your coworkers and the CEO."

"Look," I responded. "I know you're concerned about the emails. They're just thoughts, that's all. I would never hurt anyone here. I'm a nurse, for crying out loud. I don't have a criminal record."

"We're going to terminate your employment immediately. Since you haven't actually committed any crime, we won't call the police. But as someone who has known you for some time, I'd like to know if you are truly okay. Do you need to speak with a professional?"

"No, I'm okay. The funny thing is that if you saw what goes on here during the night, you'd think I'm more sane than most of the people here."

"I've never seen someone write such graphic and horrific emails. Not only are you a danger to the employees, but you are also a threat to our patients. Our guard will escort you off the premises. From this point forward you are forbidden from stepping foot on campus."

I knew I couldn't say anything for self-defense. As I walked out of the building, I realized I had made a huge mistake in writing those emails. I thought I was being smart by *not sending* them to myself. But I was an idiot for drafting the emails using my work server! As I walked into the freezing cold at 8pm, I shuttered. I didn't know what hurt more: the fact that I had just been fired again, or the fact that I couldn't feel my ears. Can you believe it was my ears?

Jobs #4 and #5

Surprisingly, my nursing career didn't end there. By applying to two jobs a day, I secured a full-time ICU gig along with a Per Diem ICU job. I knew my ICU skills were weak after spending five months in Satan's hole doing nothing. So my new goal was to stay with one nursing job for at least one year, assuming I would get fired from one of the jobs. My daily mantra became: "Someone is going to die, but I am going to live!"

I became paranoid about disciplinary action, so I became a little bitch hiding on the night shift. Sometimes I felt gay for heightening the pitch of my voice when interacting with coworkers, feigning friendliness. At other times I felt like a straight up pussy for being anal about small details, such as looking for defecation on my patients at 6am. In fact, I cleaned patients multiple times per shift just so no one would complain about me. But at least I wasn't meeting with any more VP's of Human Resources.

Five months into my two-jobbed adventure, I had not been fired from either job. I was surprised, because working two night shift jobs seriously affected my mental health. Learning from my previous gigs, I only took shortcuts when people weren't watching. I also stayed in my unit and refrained from writing emails about killing people. The fact that I was working the night shift was my lifesaver because fewer eyes were on me. Did I mention I didn't roam to other floors in search of coffee?

Sadly, the highlight of my time in the ICU was setting up a Central Venous Pressure (CVP) line. Somehow, handling different tubes and cords until I saw a squiggly line on the monitor gave my brain an orgasm. After two years of suctioning phlegm from patients' throats, giving insulin shots at 6am, and dipping my hand in diarrhea, I had finally done something that required technical skill! After stroking myself, the egoic side of me realized the sadness of the situation. Was the CVP line the only thing I could be proud of in the last two years? Sadly, it was.

After proving to myself I could hold a nursing job for at least a year, I quit both jobs in anticipation of the start of CRNA school. It seemed to be the next logical step in my career, so I decided to move forward. As I stepped onto the private school's campus, I muttered: "I bet there's no VP of Human Resources here." Little did I know that I would meet with the Dean just one year later.

CRNA School

CRNA school was a blur. I was smarter than most of the people in my class. But once the clinical portion of my program started, I couldn't hide my true nature. Because I was so used to taking shortcuts in the ICU, I automatically brought the same behavior into the OR. That is, I didn't wear gloves when touching patients, I didn't throw syringes in the proper bins, and I took shortcuts in charting. Ultimately, I got onto the administrators' radar by using a single syringe to give medications to two different patients, potentially spreading Hepatitis in the process (I didn't know my preceptor was looking at me the entire time; the night shift had made me a shortcut machine!). Oh yeah, did I mention that I created a hole in someone's mouth one week later (see chapter 5)?

The administrators put me on probation, telling me they'd kick me out if I made another mistake related to universal precautions. Needless to say, I became the gayest version of myself. I had invested too much money just to be kicked out for infection control reasons! I started acting like a little bitch, brown nosing my preceptors and giving them compliments. I was also quick to praise the anesthesiologist attendings, hoping all my supervisors would give my administrators a fine report about me. Perhaps most disgustingly, I started verbalizing my actions (*Okay, I am throwing this syringe in the proper receptacle. Please don't kick me out of the program!*).

My strategy of maximizing my gayness ultimately didn't help, because I violated infection control again. The downward spiral came on a gloomy October morning, three months after I started my probationary period. I was inserting an arterial line, which is a sterile procedure. Focused on the task and not the rules surrounding the task, I broke sterility by grabbing the packaging of the arterial line kit with my sterile gloves.

"What are you doing? You just broke the most basic step in setting up an a-line!" screamed my preceptor.

"Oops, sorry," I said.

My hands started trembling as I restarted the set up from square one. When I finally punctured the skin with the needle, I couldn't get any blood backflow. I manipulated my angle of insertion for ten minutes and still didn't get anything.

"Let me try," said the preceptor.

Frustrated, I took the needle out from under the patient's skin and threw it away. Luckily for me, I threw it away in the wrong trash bin!

"Wow, are you serious?" screamed the preceptor.

"It's not a big deal. Stop PMSing on me! I haven't compromised patient safety," I said.

The preceptor glared at me with wide eyes and unleashed herself.

"Throwing sharps away in the sharps container is a basic practice of universal precautions. Inserting an arterial line requires sterility, too. You don't even know the basic things. All nurses should be aware of these rules!"

I had nothing to say. I knew it was only a matter of time before she called my administrators, and they would know I had violated infection control procedures yet again. I spent the rest of the day in a haze. It was unbelievable that my road would come to an end because a Russian cunt caught me throwing a needle in the wrong bin. Truth be told, I thought of grabbing the needle and sticking it straight into the preceptor's throat.

"How's that for proper procedure? Hopefully I throw your body in the right bin!" I imagined myself saying.

That very afternoon, one of my administrator's asked me to take a drug screen. As I stood in the student health center's restroom with my penis in my hand, I knew my CRNA dream was over.

One week later, I was called to meet with two of the program directors, along with the Dean (I couldn't help but think my appointments with the VPs of Human Resources prepared me for this moment). I had been suspended from the OR for a week. The entire time, my gut screamed at me to prepare for the worst case and apply for nursing jobs. Did I mention that the directors wouldn't answer my calls? I guess they preferred to give disastrous news to people in person.

When I walked into the room, the director Shiza started things off.

"Walt, you are here today because you've violated universal precautions. Back in the summer, we gave you an opportunity to redeem yourself after you made two critical patient safety mistakes. However, since that time we haven't seen any improvement. Your latest infraction of universal precautions was the last straw. Because of the lack of improvement on your end, we're going to have to ask you to withdraw from the program."

"What if I were to decline?" I asked.

"Then we'd issue you a clinical dismissal. Your infractions are very basic and we feel that if you don't have the basics down at this point, then you shouldn't be allowed to progress."

Obviously, this was their way of politely kicking me out. Still, I had many questions. I had nothing to lose.

"I want to know the specific reasons I was requested to take a drug test," I said.

"We as a school have the right to request drug screens at any time. You signed a form giving us authorization."

"I want to know the specific reasons! It costs $100 for a drug screen to be analyzed. You guys are so cheap, your internet doesn't even work in this building. If you guys went that far in getting me to piss into a cup, then I want to know all the reasons. You don't expect me to believe that my throwing a needle in the wrong trash caused you guys to spend $100, do you?"

"You really want to know?"

"You guys are kicking me out, aren't you? I want to know every allegation."

"The CRNAs and attendings at the hospital no longer feel comfortable letting you give patient care. Over the past week we've received multiple complaints from many staff members, almost all of whom are experienced experts. The OR staff has complained that you routinely present to the OR without a mask, despite being told several times to wear one. They also complain that you roam the halls without a cap, and that they have caught you repeatedly without any type of head covering. You also drink water in the hallways, when that's strictly against the rules. One person even complained that she caught you staring at a wall in a disoriented state, almost as if you were hallucinating."

"I don't get why caps and masks are such a big deal. Those things have nothing to do with patient care."

"They have everything to do with patient care. Having surgeons operate in a clean environment is fundamental. And why were you staring at walls, Walt?"

"I was just thinking, that's all."

"That's only the beginning. One CRNA said that you have a tendency to walk into patient rooms with wet pants, even though he repeatedly told you not to do so."

I had a habit of putting my dick into my pants before I completely finished urinating. The wet spot was just dribbles of urine. I hoped they didn't they think I was jacking off in the restroom!

"Why are CRNAs looking at my dick?" I asked.

"That's not the point. The recurring theme has been that multiple staff members have warned you about certain actions, but you haven't listened. Also, the same CRNA complained that you are odd with patients. You completely disrobed an elderly woman to take a listen to her breath sounds, which was completely inappropriate. You are supposed to listen to breath sounds while protecting the patient's dignity."

"This is all coming from left field. What else did they moan about?"

"That you repeatedly put your knees on the floor of the hospital, despite being continuously warned against that."

I always knew I was under a microscope, but I didn't know the CRNAs would report me for such small, stupid bullshit.

"It was also reported to me that you ate other people's lunches in the nursing lounge. As a matter of fact, a Nurse Practitioner student filed a complaint saying that you stole her pizza in the classroom," Shiza continued.

"I never took anyone's lunches!"

Actually, I had taken the student's lunch because it was in the public fridge. I had later offered her ten bucks as compensation, but she refused it. So technically I never stole anything.

"Most importantly, one of the attendings said he is uncomfortable with you giving patient care. He said you have tunnel vision and aren't connecting the dots as you should be at this point. You appear frazzled and hesitate before treating patients," said Shiza.

"Actually, if you look at my performance evaluations, you'd see passing scores."

"Yes, but that doesn't negate the fact that you violated universal precautions by throwing away a needle in the wrong bin. That was a direct infraction of your probation plan."

"Any other complaints?"

"I think that's enough, don't you think?"

"I want a refund of the past year."

"That's not possible because instruction has already occurred. You got what you paid for."

I felt like I was getting raped. In my moment of loss, I wanted to come up on top, somehow.

"This is what I want from all of you," I continued. "If any program director asks about me when I apply to another school, don't reveal anything to them."

"The only intel we'll provide is your enrollment dates."

"Also, I want a letter of recommendation."

My audacity surprised even me.

"Sorry Walt, I can't do that. If I did, I'd have to reveal everything we just talked about. Walt, the fact of the matter is that the decision to let you go was unanimous among the faculty. Even if you decide not to withdraw, it would only be a matter of time before we issued you an F for your clinical grade. Plus, the hospital refused to take you back. We wouldn't be able to transfer you to another institution."

How could I win? What could I leak from them?

"I want a record of all my files, including the emails written about me," I said.

"No problem. Just send the Dean an email and she can authorize it."

"Look, the faculty views you positively," said the Dean. "You are a person of many talents. It's just that anesthesia is a very specific specialty, and it probably isn't for you. There are tons of fields in which you can potentially excel. Maybe this is an opportunity for you to find a place where the grass is greener."

"Right now, you're underperfoming," said the other director. "There's no other probation plan we can put you on. There's just not enough time for us to get you where you need to be by December."

"Ok, you'll get an email from me within a week," I said. "If you can't write me a letter, then keep your mouths shut as much as possible. I will stand back up from this. I have my youth and my health; I am still the luckiest guy in the world!" I said.

"Thanks for your optimism. That's exactly what you'll need in the next few months. In the meantime, just understand that the withdrawal form can be found online at the student homepage," said the Dean.

I stood up, gave them the finger, and bolted out the door. I ran straight to the Dean of financial aid, with whom I was on good terms.

"Bad news. They just asked me to withdraw. I need your help in getting a refund for this quarter," I said.

"Yeah, the director told me this morning. I'll get you as much as I can. Since we're halfway through the quarter, the most you can get back is fifty percent of the tuition you've already paid. The clinical fee and health insurance are nonrefundable."

I was being raped again! I wouldn't have any of it.

"I want to negotiate. Who's the ultimate decision maker? There's gotta be a guy we can call."

"That's me."

"I ask that you cut me some slack. I heard that you gave a full refund to a CRNA student last quarter when she took a leave."

"That's because her grandmother died. I give exceptions to people whose family members have passed away."

It was time to use some strategies of influence.

"I'm not going to lie and say that my grandmother died. If you're going to make exceptions, then I ask that you make an exception for me. I ask that you give me half the health insurance fee and half the clinical fee, since I'll be withdrawing midway through the quarter."

"Mmm, sorry I can't do that."

"Then at least give me half the clinical fee. I won't be showing up to the hospital for the latter half of this quarter, so I think that's fair."

"Okay fine! You'll get half the clinical fee."

I smiled. I wasn't going to get fucked while laying down. They'd see me sink with a fighting spirit.

As I left the nursing building, I realized a dream was shattered. It was time to lick my wounds, secure another job, and prepare for a long drive home.

####

Lesson One: **Follow your gut. If you think you're going to get fired, then start applying for other jobs immediately.** When the ax falls in nursing, it falls very quickly. When I was in CRNA school, I knew the faculty liked me, but I also knew I had made huge mistakes in terms of infection control. When I was requested to take a drug test and was suspended for a second time from clinicals, my gut screamed at me: "it's over." The lesson here is to not hang on to hope just because you think your overseers like you. When the shit hits the fan in your career, all you have to do is listen to your gut.

Action step: practice listening to your gut, or the visceral feeling you get about people and situations. Have you ever talked with a detestable girl? It's likely your gut screamed: "get this bitch away from me!" The very same gut feeling will be activated if you get into trouble. The way you practice listening to your gut is by paying attention to your breathing, the inflow and outflow of your breath. Only then can you bypass your racing thoughts to get at what *your body* is trying to say.

Lesson Two: **Taking shortcuts is okay to do on the night shift. But be careful on the day shift.** Am I saying that you can only take shortcuts at night? Absolutely not! I'm just telling you to be careful during the day, because that's when the administrative team is awake. There are three main shortcuts people take during the night shift. First, people routinely falsify documentation such as vital signs, nursing assessments, and medication administration times. Second, some guys cheat when it comes to cleaning patients. Not only do they NOT give baths, but they also refuse to change chucks and other types of bedding. Third, people refuse to give medications if they know the consequences will suck. For example, nurses may refuse to give laxatives because they don't want to wipe shit during their shifts. It's possible to get away with these infractions on the night shift because there's less supervision. If you're thinking of shortcutting on the day shift, just be warned: a lot more eyes will be on you.

Action step: the next time you're about to take a shortcut, ask yourself: "who is watching me right now? Are there any cameras in the room?"

Lesson Three: **If you need to get another job, make contact with the hiring manager of each unit.** This is how a loser applies for jobs: he submits his resume/cover letter using a company's hiring portal. He then waits for three months and never gets a call or email. He then wonders what he did wrong. The reality is that he only did one percent of all that he could have done.

The key to getting a job is *personally establishing contact with the hiring manager*. I'm specifically referring to the unit manager/director, not the HR recruiter or spokesperson. Remember: the only person you care about in the job hunt is the one making the decisions. All other people, including secretaries and charge nurses, are secondary in your mission. In total, there are three steps in getting a job. First, submit your resume/cover letter *using key words in the online job description*. Second, immediately call and email the hiring manager. Your goals are to introduce yourself and present an upbeat, enthusiastic attitude (think about a gay person smiling and dialing; you should pretend to be this gay person while writing emails and making calls). The way to find these managers' contact information is to call hospitals' directories and just ask for emails and numbers. If this fails, you'll just have to use google. Third, show up to the interview. Thousands of articles have been written about how to ace interviews. All I have to say is that the hiring manager will make his decision within the first 30 seconds of meeting you, so practice your smile and firm hand shake.

99% of your job hunting results will come from emailing/calling directors. Your goal should be to submit at least one job application per day, establishing contact with each hiring manager for every resume you submit. If you don't get any responses, keep smiling and dialing. It doesn't have to take three to four months to find another job. All it takes is two to four weeks.

Action step: use a single sheet of paper to capture your job leads. For each job application you submit, write down the contact information of the hiring manager. Record the dates and times of all emails, calls, and voicemails sent. Leave your footprint! Get on the radar! Leave your bodily stains every three days until you get a job interview. What do you have to lose? It's better to be annoying than jobless.

Lesson Four: **Don't create stories about getting fired.** When I first got fired at 24, catastrophic thoughts flooded my head. This is what my thinking looked like: "My career is over. No one will want to hire me. I am incompetent!" Looking back, I realize that my mind was creating stories about a single event: getting let go. I would have been healthier emotionally if I had just allowed getting fired to mean just one thing: getting fired. That is to say, my catastrophic thinking at age 24 was my mind creating stories. Getting fired is getting fired. Saying anything else about that event is your mind creating stories about something that should be left alone.

Action step: if you get subjected to disciplinary action/counseling, then write down each inciting event on a piece of paper. Record next to each event the lessons you've learned. Once this exercise is done, commit yourself to only thinking about the inciting events when necessary. Refrain from creating stories in your mind about your career prospects, intelligence, or personality.

Lesson Five: **All you have to do is follow the procedure.** If you look at the reasons my CRNA school wanted me to withdraw, you'll see that I violated proper procedures. If I had just followed the rules, I would have been fine. When I was a student, I thought some rules were so small I could get away with violating them, but the reality was that all the staff members were watching me. Remember: *the small stuff counts too.*

To sum up, follow your gut if you feel the need to apply to other jobs. Be careful when taking shortcuts on the day shift. Make contact with the gatekeepers for each job you apply to. If you get fired, don't create stories about the event. All you have to do is follow the procedure, even if it's for a small thing (like drinking water in the hallways).

Chapter 7: Dipping Your Hand In Shit

I was 22 years old and eager to get my hands wet with nursing experience. I had spent the last three years in classrooms taking endless tests. Now it was time to learn something useful!

My first unit was a general medical/surgical floor with extremely sick patients. As the charge nurse toured the students, I couldn't believe how many tubes, drains, and fluids I saw. The moans and groans weren't too reassuring, either.

One patient in room seven opened my eyes. Both the patient's arms were amputated, and he was having seizures at random times. Since he had just had surgery, he had multiple holes in his abdomen with tubes draining fluid from his intestines. To make matters worse, he had uncontrollable diarrhea. Imagine a disabled, seizing man showering people with his loose, foul stool. Then imagine him doing it at random times. Guess what? I didn't have to imagine it.

I collected myself and met up with the other students. Clearly, everyone was nervous. Cindy was breathing hard. Cynthia was blinking uncontrollably. Sally looked as if she were about to cry. I paid attention to the sounds and smells of the unit. Patient call bells were ringing off the hook, and the nurses were running around like ants. Family members were complaining. And the nursing students were huddled together, looking like they were on death row.

The instructor came late. Bich, aka the drill sergeant, was a man who coincidentally had a vagina.

"I better not get the guy in room seven," I thought.

"Walt, you'll be helping Cher, who has the patients in rooms six and seven."

"I'd actually prefer the patient in room five for the pathophysiological challenge."

"Nice try. You have six and seven."

I bit my tongue and tried to find Cher, a Korean quickster specifically chosen to handle me. Not only was I given the toughest patients, but I also had no idea what to do. I was a fish suddenly caught in a net.

"I propose that I start giving the meds for Mr. Lee in room six. I'm pretty comfortable doing it," I said.

"How about starting with Mr. Stool in room seven. His diarrhea has been heavy and we need help cleaning him up," said Cher.

I wanted to challenge her, but since I was a nursing student I was at the bottom of the totem pole. Even volunteers had it better than I did (at least they weren't paying tuition).

When I arrived in the patient's room, Mr. Stool stared at me with his mouth wide open and his tongue sticking out.

"He's friendly, don't worry," said Cher.

The odor was unbearable. It smelled like someone had raped 10 skunks and stuck them up Mr. Stool's rectum. His diarrhea was so severe that his scrotum was almost bleeding. He seemed to be saying: "lick my ass; you are my new bitch."

Like clockwork, Mr. Stool had a nice, leaky bowel movement as I walked toward him. The stool was an unearthly mix of green and yellow, the likes of which you only dream about. And it just kept coming out, intensifying the foul odor. I began to gag.

"I've already gotten the cleaning materials for you. I'd suggest you put some toothpaste and a mask on to help hide the stench."

"Am I going to get any help?"

"Yes, Carmen is our assistant today. Here's her number."

After giving me the info, Cher moved to the next patient. I frantically called Carmen, who wasn't picking up the phone. I went outside, explored the unit, and found her taking care of the diarrhea of another patient.

"Carmen, can I get your help with room seven?"

"I'm busy! And I have three other patients after this one."

I came back to my pimp, who seemed to be smirking at this point. Swallowing my pride, I gathered some wipes and cleaning fluid. I applied toothpaste to a mask, put it on my face, and noticed that foul odor was still alive and strong. I had never wiped the ass of another man before.

"There's a first time for everything. Alright my friend, it's you and me," I told my pimp.

I pushed the patient onto his side, exposing his tender buttocks. As I grabbed a towel and aimed for the anus, Mr. Stool left out a huge fart, splashing diarrhea all over my face. A nice little chunk entered my right eye. Shrieking with panic, I ran to the sink.

Mr. Stool began to seize and shake uncontrollably. The stool splashed over the bed and onto the floor.

I cleared out my eyes and tried to remain calm. I then put towels on the floor to hide the stool. Luckily for me, Cher had placed some buckets in the corner in case Mr. Stool had too much fun. I grabbed the buckets and cupped (with my bare hands) the stool on the bed into the bucket. Mr. Stool started seizing a little harder.

"I need some help in here!" I yelped.

Amazingly, no one came. Was I getting punked? Was this a rite of passage I was supposed to face on my own? I was having serious doubts about the nursing world. At the same time, I couldn't let my emotions get the best of me. Bich demanded professional behavior at all times and held the keys to progression to the next rotation.

After twenty minutes of playing with Mr. Stool's shit, I finally had the room contained and decently cleaned. Carmen came in and helped me change the patient's linens and hospital gown.

I moved on to Mr. Lee, hoping he had good sphincter control. After practically bathing myself in someone else's stool, I was about to lose my temper and had even turned red. Cher fed the fire some more.

"Mr. Lee needs a sponge bath," she said.

"How about you give it to him with me?" I replied.

"Okay, I'll be there in a few minutes."

Walking into room six, I found a 21 year old man with severe depression. Fred Lee was a PhD student who had tried to stab himself to death. He had knife wounds in the abdomen, chest, and legs. He was also on five different antidepressants.

"Hi Mr. Lee, I'm Walt. I'm here to give you a sponge bath."

Fred grinned.

I had never given a man a sponge bath before. I reluctantly wet a sponge and began gliding it over Fred's body. Fred was apparently having the time of his life, letting out pleasurable moans here and there. As I took off the patient's pants and washed the thigh area, I noticed Fred's small boner.

"Okay...where the heck is Cher?" I muttered.

I was a 22 year old guy giving a sponge bath to a 21 year old dude, who apparently couldn't get enough of the bath. As I kept moving, the doubts increased within. Was I really going to study so hard in school just to give 21 year old guys sponge baths?

All of a sudden, Fred urinated into the air, flooding my right eye. I cursed and flew straight to the sink. I was only two hours into the shift! Because diseases like Hepatitis B could be transmitted through bodily fluids, I became paranoid. First, someone had defecated in my eye. Now, someone else had urinated into the same eye. I would need to double check on the patients' histories to see if they could have infected me.

I quickly finished Fred's sponge bath. When I went back to the main hall, I had visibly aged. My eyes were red, my clothes reeked of bodily fluids, and I could barely contain myself. Not only had I been humiliated, but I was also running on an empty stomach. Thinking I could last for the entire shift, I had not brought any money to cover myself. I could feel the world weighing on my shoulders as my vision of nursing shattered in front of me. Was this what nursing was all about? Giving medications and getting crapped on?

I had no choice but to toil throughout the rest of the day. True to Cher's word, the staff nurses worked me like a dog. At the end of the day, I had spent his entire shift cleaning patients. I had been defecated on, pissed on, and vomited on. Walking home that night, I wondered how else I could be disillusioned in the months to come.

####

Lesson One: **The first time you wipe a man's ass will be overwhelming. You will feel like quitting nursing the entire day.** After my first ass-wiping session, I condemned myself and started personalizing the job of nursing. For instance, I'd ask myself: "How did I get into this mess? I got a 2200 on the SAT, so how have I descended to this level of dipping my hand in shit? I'm a failure for sucking this badly at life." Notice that I created a story (and an identity) from the simple act of cleaning a patient. That is, *I created a negative interpretation of an event.* In turn, this negative interpretation lowered my self-esteem and ultimately made me leave nursing. If I had just let the event be without creating any stories, I would have suffered less.

Action step: The next time you wipe another man's ass, smile and notice your negative thoughts (if they occur). Let them drift away without creating any stories in your head about your worth as a human being. Your job is your job...move on.

Lesson Two: **Have fun with the different smells you encounter.** Is it miserable to wipe diarrhea in an ICU? Yup. Will you cry inside when you have to wipe diarrhea multiple times for different patients? Of course! That said, there's a way to have fun. Arouse your own curiosity.

Action step: when you get a good whiff of diarrhea, ask yourself what foods might have created that stench. Then, begin to wonder whose shit smells worse: yours or your patient's. If yours smell worse, pat yourself on the back. *Create curiosity from the curious smells you encounter.*

Lesson Three: **Remember that the "wiping phase" is only temporary.** Most men reading this book will only work at the bedside for a couple of years before moving on to school or a management role. If you get discouraged by your cleaning role, take solace in the fact that you will be moving on sooner or later.

To sum up, realize that the first time you wipe another man's ass will be overwhelming. Have fun with the different smells! Remember that the "wiping phase" is only temporary.

Chapter 8: How To Go To School For Free

"Dude, how are we going to pay for four years of college?" asked my brother Sark.

"It's actually going to be five, since we're changing our majors to nursing," I replied.

"The cost of tuition and living expenses is $25,000 a year. We're looking at a total bill of over $125,000!"

"Look, if Dad could do it, we can do it. I have a plan."

"Transfer to a junior college?"

"Nah, we're staying right here. Let's make this a competition. I'll bet you 500 bucks that I'll graduate with less debt than you."

"You're on."

Five years later, I graduated in the black from a school that costed over 100 grand. I was basically paid to go to school. What was the key? I didn't have a 4.0 GPA, and I didn't have a rich dad to milk. In reality, many people viewed me with contempt because of my autistic symptoms. But I never let my medical condition sway me. I was incredibly tenacious in the scholarship hunt and leveraged the rule that consistency is the only thing that matters.

After my bet, I moved with purpose and set up appointments with the Associate Dean and Director of Financial Aid at the School of

Nursing. I told them about my commitment to graduate with no debt. In turn, they agreed to send scholarship opportunities my way.

My second strategy was to build a team. I shared my goal with three friends in my nursing club, and they were touched by my debt-free vision. In turn, we formed a Mastermind Group. We sent scholarship opportunities to each other, shared advice, edited one another's drafts, and celebrated scholarship victories. By sharing a common vision in a spirit of harmony, each group member was motivated to move towards scholarship success.

Once I had established a base of scholarship opportunities, I created a rule for myself called the One Hour Rule, which required that I wake up one hour earlier than I normally would and work on scholarships for one hour straight. Upon waking, I would not check my email or even try to take a shit. I would simply draft and submit scholarship applications. By following the One Hour Rule, I made time in my schedule to balance schoolwork, my part time job, and the scholarship hunting process. More importantly, I generated a lifestyle conducive to scholarship success. After one month, the One Hour Rule was no longer just a rule; rather, it was a subconscious habit.

Along my journey, I faced many, many discouraging moments. For instance, there was a stretch where I had won no scholarships, even though I had submitted over 75 applications! I had put my heart and soul into each submission, even going to the extent of reaching out to extremely specialized scholarship programs, including one designed for Jewish women (to my credit, I asked the program if I could apply, and they agreed). Winning nothing, I felt as if my heart had been crushed. But in my darkest moments, I thought of my bet with Sark. I thought of him winning scholarships and showing off his cash to me with a huge grin. There was no way I was going to let him win! Needless to say, the competitive fire between me and Sark propelled me to take massive action on my debt-free vision despite my lack of results.

College ended up costing more than $125,000. Still, I was able to graduate with no debt. The key was my perseverance with the One Hour Rule despite my initial rut. My habits eventually generated powerful momentum, and over the course of five years I was able to cover my college costs with *money I did not have to pay back*. That said, my bet with my brother was the catalyst. My reward for following through was found not only in a $500 cash infusion from his bank account, but also in a life-changing lesson.

Financial success results from daily habits, not huge windfalls. In truth, I have won less than 10% of the scholarships to which I have ever applied. At the same time, I was able to graduate without debt because I maximized the number of my applications. Because I spent at least an hour everyday applying to scholarships, I produced real results in that facet of my life. Simply put, I learned that if one is serious about financial independence, then one must take small and tangible financial actions every day. Such experiences accumulate to produce huge results in the long term. The only requirement is consistent action.

Here's another tool I learned: if you're having fun writing your essay/story, then the scholarship judges will probably have fun reading it. The converse is also true: if you're getting bored writing your essay, then your judges will probably yawn and throw your application away. So how do you have fun doing such a horrendous task such as writing? The key is to *write for yourself*. Below is a template I created for a domestic violence organization. My goal was to make myself laugh. I actually received a cash prize for the entry.

Start of the essay:

My experiences as a victim of domestic violence have motivated me to become a nurse so I can offer psychiatric help to those in need. My journey in domestic violence began one night at the office.

"How's it hanging, big boy?" asked Candy.

"Not too well. Got tons of papers and clients. Can you lend a hand?" I replied.

"Depends on what kind of hand you're talking about."

"I can't be screwing around. I'm in a tight situation."

"Want to know what else is tight?"

"Our budget?"

Candy locked the door to my office and advanced toward me. It was seven o'clock at night, and we were the only ones in the building. Surprised by her aggression, I stood up.

"What are you doing?" I asked.

"Shut up!"

Candy pushed me onto my chair. I fought back, but she had the higher ground. Trained as a Mixed Martial Arts (MMA) fighter, Candy forced me into submission and began to take off my clothes. As I attempted to writhe my way out of her grasp, she countered with a firmer hold. Though my body was larger, her technique was superior. Eventually, I lost sensation in my arms and could not move my extremities. I could do nothing to stop her advances.

"Help!" I screamed.

It was useless. Candy tightened her hold and had her way with me.

When she was done, I was crushed. I will forever remember that night as the time my girlfriend raped me.

That night was a catalyst for the downward spiral of my physical and emotional wellness. Prior to that event, our relationship showed symptoms of domestic violence. Not only would Candy attempt to control where I went and belittle my choice of friends, but she would also threaten to hurt herself. Since both her parents had recently passed away, she wanted a sense of control in our relationship. Her self-esteem was lacking, so I began sponsoring MMA classes to give her a sense of control. I never would have imagined she would use MMA techniques to subdue me.

After my traumatic incident, I told Candy I was ending our relationship. To my surprise, she subsequently tried to commit suicide, overdosing on Tylenol. When I visited the hospital, her physician told me she had barely survived. If our neighbor had waited even 10 minutes before reporting the suicide attempt, Candy would not have made it.

As I looked at her recovering body in the hospital bed, feelings of guilt flooded my heart. I was her only resource, her only friend. I was trapped in a vicious circle of self-blame for her attempt to end her own life.

Candy eventually made a full recovery. From that point forward, the symptoms of domestic violence intensified. Candy prevented me from seeing my friends and family members. Furthermore, she spent almost all the income I was earning. Eventually, she physically prevented me from going to work. I felt powerless to leave because I knew her threats of suicide were genuine.

The last straw came when I was terminated from my job for poor attendance. At that point, I was physically, emotionally, and financially depleted. My fear of her suicide and the inevitable self-blame that would result had crippled me emotionally.

At my wits' end, I traveled 2000 miles to visit my brother, Sark. I brought only a handful of clothes and 1000 dollars in cash, desperate to reinvent myself. I relayed to Sark everything that had transpired for the last couple of years, and he responded sympathetically. With his help, I started a therapy program to recover from my clinical depression. In the beginning stages of therapy, I found out that Candy had attempted suicide again and had actually succeeded.

I was devastated. I relied on Sark to get through the next couple of months. As I had anticipated, a cycle of self-blame and guilt flooded me. The emotional trauma from Candy's suicide was consuming, but my relationships with Sark and my counselors sustained me. In all, it took three years of therapy and spiritual counseling for me to recover from my depressive episode. In fact, I continue to receive help for emotional and physical trauma. At the same time, I am committed to a full recovery.

My experiences with Candy have inspired me to help others going through relationships similar to mine. Though I stumbled emotionally after Candy's death, I have had a spiritual awakening. That said, I am committed to helping others undergoing domestic violence. By pursuing a nursing degree, I hope to empower others and advocate for vulnerable persons. Specifically, as a nurse I will help my clients uncover early warning signs of domestic violence. I hope to lend a sympathetic ear and guide my clients on their paths towards leaving caustic relationships. Ultimately, I hope to be a supportive guide and patient advocate as victims embark on their journeys toward more fulfilling lives.

Although my relationship with Candy has scarred me, it does not define me. By reinventing myself as a nurse, I hope to translate my negative experiences into positive lessons for others. In my journey of helping others undergoing domestic violence, I hope to be a ray of light, just as Sark was in my time of need. Indeed, I lived in darkness in the past, but I am recovering and am committed to showing others the light.

The End

There are two things that should scream at you: a) this story reeks of bullshit, and b) the story is extreme and therefore memorable. Other than that, the essay is an example of *incredibly bad writing*. The story is redundant and way too long. I myself lost interest halfway through once I knew what the moral of the story was going to be. But this entry still got me scholarship money because it was one heck of a story. It had drama, fantasy, suicide, sex, rape, domestic violence, and other juicy topics you just don't see in most essays. Ultimately, I was awarded for my courage, not my integrity or my writing skills. The same standards will apply to you. The ultimate lesson is that your writing doesn't have to be good to glean awards; you just need to tell entertaining stories. And the more extreme they are, the better.

Many will read this chapter and become skeptical, wondering if it's truly possible to win tens of thousands of dollars by playing the scholarship game. These are the very ones that will try my strategies for a month and then quit. However, the real audience I'm aiming for will actually try my strategies for a year and end up winning real money. For these non-quitters, my best advice is to continue to write whatever you see and hear (advice directly from Stephen King himself). I'd also add that you should go wherever the pain is. That is, write about your dark side and the mistakes that bring you the most pain and regret. You will be richly rewarded.

####

Lesson One: **Forget about working. Focus on scholarship money, which is nontaxable income.** Let's use the example of a guy called Joe. What if I were to tell Joe that in real estate, agents close sales on one in ten people they prospect? Don't you think Joe would start selling like there's no tomorrow, knowing that he'll close on 10% of his victims? Well, I'm telling you that the exact same principle applies to scholarship money. *You will win one in ten scholarships to which you apply.* This means you need to get off your couch and start applying. Is playing the scholarship game hard work? Of course it is. But it's one of the few ways to gain untaxed income.

Action Step: Sign up for scholarship databases such as unigo.com and fastweb.com, which will leak scholarship opportunities to your inbox. When it comes to scholarships, my best advice is to just get started. How do you win thousands of dollars? One application at a time.

Lesson Two: **Ritualize the behavior of applying to scholarships.** Specifically, write/hunt for scholarships every day first thing in the morning for one month. Eventually, you will get to the point where you won't even need to think. Every morning, your body will plop right in front of your computer to engage in the scholarship hunt.

Action Step: Every day in the first week of applying for scholarships, just ask yourself: "can I just write one shitty paragraph?" This question will lower the energy barrier to getting started, allowing you to initiate essay writing with low goals. Once the flow of writing kicks in, you'll write much more than one paragraph. Even if you don't get into the flow, you'll still have a shitty paragraph, which is better than nothing.

Lesson Three: **Lie your ass off by telling whacky stories.** Remember applying for colleges when you were 17 years old? Remember how you lied about being in student government and being the captain of the cross country team (the amount of lying in my high school was off the charts)? You lied with impunity because you knew the college application readers wouldn't make the effort to double check. Guess what? The exact same principle applies here. On every scholarship application, committee members have no time to verify the content of applications. They are too busy reading the sheer volume of applications. What this means for you is that you need to lie your ass off. *In fact, my experience is that even when I lied my ass off, I still only won 10% of the scholarships I applied to. That means that many of your competitors are lying sons of bitches, too.*

Action Step: Put yourself in the position of a scholarship reader. Would you want to read an essay about a guy's 3.7 GPA? Or would you rather hear a sob story about a female teenager getting gang raped by her dad, uncle, and brother at the same time? Wouldn't you start applauding if this female teenager made a commitment to become a lawyer specializing in child rape law? The bottom line is that I would give money to anyone that could make me laugh or cry. Your mission is therefore to make people laugh or cry when they read your essay. Tell a fucking story!

Lesson Four: **Write exactly what the scholarship committee wants to hear.** Scholarship committees award money for the weirdest shit. Your job is to fill their applications with the weird shit they are looking for. For instance, if you are applying for a scholarship from an autism organization, tell a story about how you have autism. *Do not write about anything else, including your GPA.* If an organization seeks to award applicants with three testicles, write an essay about your adventures in gym class being called the "tri-baller." And if the organization is looking for applicants affected by cancer, write a story about how everyone in your family has leukemia and how your mission in life is to find the cure to cancer. *The point is to tell the committee exactly what it wants to hear.* You need to adhere to this rule because scholarship committees are filled with old, saggy volunteers who want to hear a good story. Give them what they want, and they will give you untaxed money. If you tell outlandish stories and still don't receive scholarships, the worst case scenario is that you won't win any money. In that case, you will be in the same boat as the rest of your lazy classmates who settle for student loans. *You have nothing to lose...now write a story!*

Action step: after finishing any application, re-read your work while pretending to be the president of the scholarship committee. Ask yourself if you would give money to the applicant.

Lesson Five: **In the first sentence of your essay, answer the prompt. From the second sentence onward, just tell a story.** Don't get too cute by dedicating an entire paragraph to answering essay prompts. That's the quickest way to put your scholarship reader (who is already dozing off) to sleep. Instead, just answer the essay question and go for the kill with an extreme story (that'll wake them up!). How extreme should your story be? Let's just put it this way: I *am dying* to hear a good story. Even if I know you're bullshitting me, I will award you if you can put a smile on my face.

Lesson Six: **Your scholarship essay should make the reader laugh out loud or cry like a little bitch. Either way, the reader should be on the floor in the fetal position after reading your application.** That is to say, don't be boring!

Action step: after you finish any essay, have a friend read it. Ask your crony if he laughed or cried. If he didn't, then edit your draft until your crony laughs or cries (preferably in the fetal position).

Lesson Seven: **You will go through a period of three to six months where you win nothing. You will get discouraged, but keep plugging away.** Most people quit after the first month because they get no results. They would rather get a part time job for the peace of mind a paycheck brings. In so doing, they sacrifice the tens of thousands of dollars of untaxed income that only patience and consistency can bring in the scholarship game. Do yourself a favor: commit to the scholarship process everyday for at least one year. *This means drafting and submitting scholarship applications every single day for at least 30 minutes, charting your time logged every day so you can see if you're actually executing the process.* As your applications get rejected, reach out to the scholarship organizations and ask for feedback. As you continually refine your essays, you'll start creating templates for common essay prompts. Eventually, you'll win money due to the law of large numbers (remember that you'll win 10% of the ones you submit). Your awards will implicitly tell you which templates actually work (the ones that bring in the dough). By tailoring and submitting your winning templates for each scholarship application, you will amplify the amount of money you win without an increase in effort. Eventually, it may only take you one hour to apply for a scholarship, since you'll be recycling past templates. After the first six months, your winnings should keep accumulating.

What if you fall into a situation where you've been writing and submitting applications for six months and still haven't won anything? This is called hitting rock bottom, and 99% of people quit at this point. My advice in this situation is to not quit. Once you give up in the scholarship game, you ensure that people, who have no advantage other than persistence, will enjoy scholarship revenue while you cry in bed a quitter. The true winners in the game set up rituals and stick with them for at least a year. When the winners get discouraged, depressed, or mentally stuck, they just stick to the system. Motivation is fleeting, but systems and rituals don't fail.

Action step: in the beginning, focus on small scholarships worth 250-500 bucks. It may take an entire week to complete your first scholarship application. That said, this time-consuming process is a type of revenue in itself, because the beginning stages are the template-creating stages.

To sum up, focus on the scholarship hunt as a student rather than the work grind. Ritualize the behavior of applying to scholarships. Lie your ass off! Write exactly what they want to hear. Start your essays off by immediately answering the essay questions, followed by a story. Your essay should make readers laugh or cry. Keep plugging away.

Chapter 9: How To Leave Nursing And Get Owned

It had been a couple of months since I had finished nursing school, and I hadn't taken my boards yet. I thought I was too good (and way too smart) to be a nurse. I decided to try a career in sales because my college's career center spit out some results saying I'd be great at selling life insurance.

A week later I found myself in a sales office with a glorious view of downtown. I turned around in my expensive chair. Thirty feet across my desk were a couple of 40 year old secretaries, well over the hill. They were used up, fat, and probably eggless. I wondered how a 23 year old (like myself) could deserve to work in a lofty office while people twice my age could be working outside in cubicles. What was the catch?

A black sales manager walked into my office.

"Smile and dial, rookie. SMILE AND DIAL!" he yelled.

The truth hit me like a pissed off girlfriend. The secretaries had job security, while I had a quota to meet as a life insurance salesman. The office space was a nice way of telling me *you only get to stay if you sell, bitch!*

I stood up, jumped up and down to get myself in state, and grinned like the Grinch.

"YEAHHHH!" I screamed.

I was feeling the power! Blood rushed into my pale hands as I started my mantra.

"I am the greatest salesman in the world! The life insurance I sell is full of life, vitality, and superiority! I am a fucking magnet!!"

I grabbed the phone and dialed the 50th number on my spreadsheet. I smiled the entire time. For the 50th time that day, it went straight to voicemail.

"Hi! This is Walt from Cigna! Our company just revamped our life insurance portfolio, and I would love to open a conversation with you about it. I would also love to develop a close and intimate relationship with you based on trust. You can reach me back at 818-900-9172. Please call me back!" I heartily said.

I was feeling the flow, just like Tony Robbins said I would. I looked up the 51st number, smiled my ass off, and dialed again. Another white man's voicemail greeted me. I repeated my opening line, sounding gayer than a homosexual dude in a dildo factory.

As soon as I hung up, I realized I had reached the end of the broker list. It was time to re-start from the top. Maybe I could catch these guys right after lunch?

"Hi, this is Walt from Cigna! I am calling you again to let you know that my company just gave me special permission to give you a discount on our group insurance rates. I want to develop a trusting relationship with you! I would be excited to get to know you better. You can reach me at 818-900-9172. Have an EXCELLENT and WONDERFUL day!" I ejaculated.

The cold calling (and cold lies) went on and on until I got sick of hearing my own voice.

"Just pick up the phone, and I will come right over and suck your dick!" I imagined myself saying.

What a brutal job! I had been smiling and dialing since 8am, but not one broker had picked up the phone. It was now 3pm, so the only thing I could do was send emails. As I smiled and typed, my face started hurting. The next step was dropping by insurance houses on a whim. If these brokers didn't pick up the phone, maybe they'd respond to a knock on the door.

Sure enough, two weeks later I was on the road. I had been assigned to Essex County (aka the Wyoming of the United States), where farmers engaged in bestiality and the white man reigned supreme. My mission: sell life insurance to 40 year old Caucasians. Mission impossible!

I barely had any experience with white people and wanted to know the type of things they talked about. I studied films with Tom Cruise and Tom Hanks, the most Caucasian guys out there. I even looked up baseball, snowboarding, and golf just in case the brokers wanted to bullshit with me. By filling myself with the type of stuff white people liked, I hoped to be the whitest Indian in America.

Mr. Cruz, a chubby Caucasian in his mid forties, was the first broker on my list. I walked into Mr. Cruz's room with my chest out, forcing a smile and hoping I didn't look like a pedophile.

"Cigna's next sucker has arrived!" said Mr. Cruz.

"I've been sucking on this life insurance Mr. Cruz, and it sure tastes good!" I said.

"Excellent! It's been a year since Cigna sent a salesman here. I was beginning to get worried."

"They take their time in searching for the best."

"They also never change their strategy. They always delegate the shitty territories to the rookies. I'm guessing you have Essex County? You will be burning gas all day!"

"Essex is mine, sir."

"The only way you will succeed is if your rates are low. You Cigna guys are notorious for your high rates. That's why all the sales guys quit after six months."

That was news to me. No wonder I was only one of two salesmen in the office.

"Our rates may be high, but I will be responsive to your needs and answer all questions with integrity," I said. It was the only thing I could think of.

"That's what they always say before they quit. I'll be honest with you, kid. I do business with a few guys who sell both health and life insurance. You are at a huge disadvantage because you only sell life insurance. Even though you have some disability insurance on the side, no one cares because there's no money in disability. You probably won't be around much longer, kid. What did you study in college?"

"Nursing."

"Nursing! I know a couple of kids who'd die to get into that field. I heard it's tough to get a spot as a student. Why the heck are you selling insurance?"

"I don't like nursing, sir. The smell of patients nauseates me."

"At least there's job security in health care. With your sales gig, the odds of getting axed are incredible. At the very least, you should get your RN license."

"I appreciate the advice. But I'm intent on succeeding in this sales role. Will you give me a chance?"

"Send me your Request for Proposal and I'll see if your prices have come down."

Mr. Cruz called me a week later and laughed out loud. Cigna's rates had actually increased! *Stick to nursing, kid.*

After thousands of voicemails, two appointments, and zero sales, I quit the job. I found myself six months post graduation with no nursing job and no nursing license. Even though I hated nursing, I knew I had to go back. At the very least, I'd have some job security and wouldn't have to drive to no man's land, only to be rejected by 40 year old men. It appeared that I had two choices: either clean 40 year old men, or try to sell life insurance to them.

"Fuck insurance. I will smile and clean," I said to myself as I sat down for the nursing boards.

####

Lesson One: **A JOB will make you want to Jump Off a Bridge (hence the term "job").** Most jobs suck. Twenty year olds have a tendency to believe that once they start making money, life will be so much easier. Such thoughts translate into fantasies of perfect jobs. However, the truth is that most jobs *suck*. If you ever find yourself resenting nursing or feeling you're too smart to be cleaning patients, just remember that any other job would probably suck just as much. As a matter of fact, jobs in other fields would probably suck even more than a job in nursing, since nursing offers incomparable job security.

Action step: Imagine yourself miserable/stressed out in nursing. You are hungry, thirsty, and feel that you could have done so much more with your life. Then, imagine my voice telling you: "this is a JOB. It will make you want to Jump Off a Bridge! What did you expect, buddy?"

Lesson Two: **The key to happiness in healthcare is to manage your expectations. Lower the bar!** I initially left nursing because I was profoundly disappointed. I hated how I had to listen to female superiors who were clearly dumber than me. I also resented listening to doctors and feeling that I was at the bottom of the healthcare ladder. I decided to leave nursing in the second month of my ICU preceptorship when recurring thoughts of "I should just kill myself" flooded my head whenever my alarm rang. Looking back, I realize the source of my disappointment was my sky-high expectations of nursing. If I had just expected my time in nursing to be unimpressive, I would have hedged against disappointment.

Action step: during your drive to your shift, repeat the following phrase: "today will probably suck, but I will persist with patience over time."

Lesson Three: **You will be curious about what a corporate job feels like. For the most part, corporate jobs are meaningless.** An office job sounds nice and easy! You won't have to deal with blood, feces, or urine. Just remember, though, that if you're working in a corporate job it may suck your soul dry. After all, if you're not sending needless emails, then you're pushing papers or attending stupid meetings. However, in nursing you are actually helping people. The reality is that you are simply a cog in the wheel whether you work in healthcare or the corporate world. But at least in health care, you deliver value to the people you serve.

Action step: Whenever you're talking with friends about your jobs, pay attention to the words the people with desk jobs use. Ask your friends what kind of value they create in the world. When their answers disappoint you, go ahead and smile.

Lesson Four: **No matter how you feel, take the nursing boards and become a Registered Nurse once you graduate**. When I was in sales, I met a 30 year old blonde selling insurance. She had graduated at 23 with a nursing degree, but she never took the board exam. The sad thing was that we were both about to get axed cause we hadn't sold anything for five months. Here's the lesson: when you inevitably feel that you are too good to be a nurse, you will be tempted to walk away from the field. You may want to finish your relationship with nursing by defiantly refusing to take the nursing board exam. *If you don't take the nursing boards, you will regret it for the rest of your life.* It was only when I quit my sales job that I realized that job security as a nurse is priceless.

Action step: When your school administrators give you details on how to sign up for your nursing boards, *take immediate action.* Before that day ends, take the first step, whether that be creating an online account or signing up for your school's test prep class.

Lesson Five: **Don't be embarrassed about the work of nursing.** Ever see a male nurse who was excellent at his job? Ever notice how your respect for him skyrocketed? You can be that all-star male nurse who impresses patients and family members. But it all starts with respecting your position and your role in the healthcare field.

Action step: as you go about your work day, make an active effort to smile more. By pretending to be proud and acting happy, you will become proud and happy. *You become whoever you pretend to be.*

To sum up, most jobs suck. Lower your expectations. Corporate jobs suck even more. Take your nursing boards right when you are eligible! And don't be embarrassed to be a nurse.

Chapter 10: The Sunk Cost Fallacy

When I was 18, I told myself to become a CRNA. Seduced by the mysterious gas-giving people working behind the scenes, I committed myself to this career. Starting at 19, I emailed the directors of the nurse anesthesia programs in New York, requesting guidance on how to be admitted (if it sounds like ass licking, it's because that's what it was). My early twenties were spent taking CRNA school prerequisites, studying for the GRE, and vying for an ICU job just to position myself as an ideal candidate. I remember crying at 22 because I wanted to be CRNA so much! I was sad because I had gotten an A- in a science class and thought my chances of getting admitted had been jeopardized.

It took eight years to get my undergraduate degree and the critical care experience needed to apply to CRNA schools. Not surprisingly, I was admitted on my first try to two out of the three schools (one of them rejected me because they thought I was really intense...fuck them!). Little did I know that I'd be forced to withdraw just one year later. As I drove home that night, I knew I had two choices: I could either persist and try to get into another CRNA program, or I could quit my CRNA dream.

What made my decision tough was the fact that my CRNA dream had taken ten years of my life. I had studied my tail off, competing against pre-med students in the raw sciences. I had volunteered at the medical center and gotten to know the managers to optimize my chances of getting a new grad ICU position in a teaching hospital. I had also gotten multiple certifications just to appear sexy in front the the CRNA program committees. I had even tolerated three years on the night shift, losing out on the prime years of my life just so I could qualify for school. In my early and mid twenties, there were no girlfriends, very few night outs, and even fewer sexual experiences along the way (there were very few hours of sleep, too).

I ultimately quit the CRNA dream because I realized I was following the dreams of an 18 year old kid. All my planning and orchestrating stemmed from the cunning of a teenager, and I was still prone to listening to him! I also realized I had no passion for giving anesthesia. More importantly, I quit the CRNA dream because I realized I'd be falling prey to the sunk cost fallacy by persisting.

If you were in Vegas and had lost $10,000 at a blackjack table, would you keep playing? Most people would keep going in an attempt to recover their losses, which is the typical behavior of people suffering from the sunk cost fallacy. They have been conditioned toward loss aversion and find it unbearable to live with great losses, so they convince themselves to keep playing with the hope that they'll win money in the ensuing rounds. However, the logical thing to do would be to walk away from the table. Indeed, even lower life forms, including small children, show a tendency to walk away from events that have created pain in the past. Responsible adults could learn a thing or two. That is, if an event sucks and causes pain, then walk away. Lower life forms have taught us that by avoiding the sunk cost fallacy, we can create our futures, rather than repeat the mistakes of the past.

Metaphorically speaking, I was in Vegas at the age of 28. I had lost $10,000 (representing time and money) pursuing my CRNA dream. My emotions screamed at me to keep playing the CRNA game in order to justify my losses. But my logical side realized I should just walk away before I lost even more resources and time to a dream of an 18 year old kid. Was it painful to realize I was walking away from ten years of work? Hell yes! But I viewed my future outside the CRNA realm to be more desirable than my life within the CRNA bubble. I executed accordingly.

When I moved back home to my parents' house at the age of 28, I realized the upcoming year would really suck. I'd have to pay off $30 grand of debt from CRNA school and figure out what to do with my nursing career. But at the very least, I'd be able to create a future independent of the past faulty decisions I had made.

####

Lesson One: **In your twenties, it will seem that everyone will want to go back to school to get their MSN or CRNA credential. Don't listen to the noise.** In fact, I recommend delaying graduate school until you are 26-28 years old. It is only in this age range that a man begins to see how complex a human life can get. A man's ability to exercise self-control isn't fully intact until he reaches that age, as well. If you do enroll in graduate school before the age of 26, there's a good chance you're doing it because of peer pressure. You've been warned!

Lesson Two: **Don't stick to a career path simply because you chose it at 18 years of age.** When you reach 26-28, I'd recommend re-evaluating the reasons you are on your career track. If any of the reasons have anything to do with your plans at the age of 18, then you need to re-consider your motives. Are you being driven by a yearning to be great at what you do? Or are you being driven by the plans of a younger version of yourself? Only you know that answer.

Lesson Three: **If you ever doubt your career path while in graduate school or beyond, ask yourself what a little kid would do in your situation.** Remember how I said lower life forms make decisions, taking account if something has caused them previous pain? That is exactly what you should do! In other words, don't persist in a career path simply because you fear the losses you'd incur by walking away. Instead, act like a child. That is, make decisions and be willing to incur losses so you can create a brighter future for yourself. Be willing to quit what clearly is not working.

To sum up, don't listen to the noise of people clamoring to get back to school. Don't stick to a career path simply because you chose it in your youth. If you start having doubts, ask yourself what a little kid would do.

The Last Page

If you laughed at all, I only ask one thing: leave a review for my book on amazon.com. My goal in life is to help nurses express themselves freely so they can have power in their lives and in the workplace.

You can reach me at nursewaltcummings@gmail.com if you have questions or comments.

Visit my site at malenurseblog.com for more stories/commentary on the nursing profession.

www.ingramcontent.com/pod-product-compliance
Lightning Source LLC
Chambersburg PA
CBHW021500210526
45463CB00002B/818